The
Get With
the
Program!
GUIDE TO
FAST FOOD
and
FAMILY
RESTAURANTS

BOB GREENE

SIMON & SCHUSTER
New York   London   Toronto   Sydney

With special thanks to Daryn Eller
for her contribution to this work.

SIMON & SCHUSTER
Rockefeller Center
1230 Avenue of the Americas
New York, NY 10020

First Simon & Schuster trade paperback edition 2004

SIMON & SCHUSTER and colophon are registered trademarks
of Simon & Schuster, Inc.

MAKE THE CONNECTION and GET WITH THE
PROGRAM are registered trademarks of Harpo, Inc.

For information regarding special discounts for
bulk purchases, please contact
Simon & Schuster Special Sales at 1-800-456-6798 or
business@simonandschuster.com

Designed by Helene Berinsky

Manufactured in the United States of America

10 9 8 7 6 5 4 3 2 1

Library of Congress Cataloging-in-Publication Data
Greene, Bob.
    The get with the program! guide to fast food and
family restaurants / Bob Greene.
        p. cm.
    1. Fast food restaurants—United States—Guidebooks.
    2. Restaurants—United States—Guidebooks.
    3. Nutrition. I. Title.

TX907.2.G76 2004
647.9573—dc22   2003066657

ISBN 0-7432-5621-2

The
Get With
the
Program!
GUIDE TO
FAST FOOD
and
FAMILY
RESTAURANTS

Introduction

I've always loved eating in restaurants: I take great pleasure in the artful cooking (and sometimes even the not-so-artful cooking) of others. But to be honest, in recent years I've eaten out more than I'd really like to. Because I travel so much, dining out is often more a matter of necessity than of choice, making me feel somewhat like a prisoner of someone else's menu. There's no doubt that it's harder to eat healthfully at restaurants than at home; you have less control over the choices available and how food is prepared, and it's harder to tell if what you think you're eating is what you're *really* eating—and harder to put the brakes on temptation.

But, if you approach dining out with the same amount of knowledge and commitment you bring to eating at home, there's no reason you can't eat out *and* stay on the program, whether you go to restaurants once, twice, thrice, or many more times a week.

This is even more true today than it was just a short while ago. All the traveling I've done over the past few years has given me the opportunity to sample restaurants in almost every nook and cranny of the country, and I think I can say with some authority that the state of restaurant food is improving. The management of many eateries, from four-star dining rooms to fast-food joints, seems to have heard the cry for more healthful entrees—and they're delivering. Restaurants, after all, are businesses, and many health-conscious people have dollars to spend. I'm sure that there are some restaurateurs out there who have changed their menus because they have a social conscience (and probably like to eat nutritious food themselves), but, for the most part, the bottom line being the bottom line in business, it's our dollars that are driving the market.

Just a few years ago, healthy restaurant fare wasn't particularly marketable. Some places tried putting a few nutritious options onto their menus but no one bought them. Now, though, people are responding to these healthier choices, partly, I think, because restaurant chefs have learned to make them much more palatable. For example, at the time of this writing, McDonald's had recorded a significant jump in overall sales that analysts attributed to the introduction of a line of salads called Premium Salads. Wendy's and Jack in the Box have also introduced new and improved salads of their own. Many chains are putting considerable energy into getting across the news that fast-food restaurants now offer healthier choices. I know this firsthand because (in the interest of full disclosure) I have even been hired as a consultant to help McDonald's with its healthy lifestyles public awareness campaign.

But it's not just fast-food restaurants that are getting into the act; all kinds of places are now much more open to special requests (that is, the waiter no longer makes you feel like crawling under the table when you ask for salad dressing on the side). Many sit-down restaurants, from coffee shops to four-star dining rooms, have even created special dishes for those of us concerned about the condition of our arteries and how our jeans fit. In doing the research for this book, I was also amazed at how many restaurants post nutritional analyses of their food on their Web sites. Doing a little Web surfing before you dine out is really worth the time.

All this is good news, but restaurants are still far from perfect, and because they're not it's still important to approach dining out with caution and intelligence. Researchers have found that there is a direct connection between the frequency with which people eat out and the amount they weigh, and this is particularly true of fast-food dining: The more people eat out at fast-food restaurants, the more extra pounds they tend to carry. Plus, not all the recent changes in restaurant menus have been made with your health in mind. There has been, for instance, a movement by restaurants (particularly, though not exclusively, fast-food restaurants) to supersize just about everything. Suddenly we're facing dishes with modifiers such as "monster" and "towering," not to mention employees trying to get you to upsize "for just a quarter more." It may be a good deal financially speaking, but healthwise I can't think of a worse investment.

It's easy to get angry at the restaurant industry for what might be seen as an assault on our health and the promotion of obesity. And many people *have* gotten angry—so angry that they've brought lawsuits intending to make restaurants (fast-food restaurants especially) pay for feeding us poorly. I prefer to look at it a different way. We can all make choices, and that includes choosing whether to buy the supersize fries or the small-size fries—or, better yet, a plain baked potato or a side salad. We can also choose not to eat everything on our plate. If being wasteful is a concern, well, all restaurants carry doggy bags or some other type of take-home container.

These days, thanks to the health messages kids get in school, public service messages on TV, and news reports on nutrition, it's the rare person who doesn't know at least the basics of eating right. We all have a pretty good idea that living exclusively on French fries, hamburgers, and shakes is not healthy. And we all know that a monster cola is going to have far more calories than a small cup of soda (and that water is a far better selection). It's the personal responsibility of each and every one of us to make the right choices. It's our responsibility at the grocery store and at home, and it shouldn't be any different when we dine out.

There is no doubt that restaurants continually put temptation in our paths, but this is where your commitment to yourself comes in. In *Get With the Program* and *The Get With the Program! Guide to Good Eating,* I laid out choices intended to set you on a path toward a stronger, healthier body and an improved life. I hope that at this point (with or without the help of those two books) you have committed to three steps that will lead you to success:

- Becoming stronger and healthier through exercise
- Getting a grip on emotional eating
- Maintaining a nutritious diet

I think that once you've committed yourself to reaching those goals, it will make it easier to extend your commitment to restaurant dining. Staying on the program in the face of alluring double cheeseburgers and pasta in cream sauces takes inner strength, but if you've been working hard to eat well and exercise, you already have what it takes to tackle the obstacles restaurants menus put in your path.

What will also help you stay the course is beginning to think about restaurant dining in a new way. People dine out for different reasons. Sometimes it's for a social occasion or a celebration, sometimes it's simply to sample the latest hot spot. Sometimes it's a business obligation or, as in my case, because travel leaves you no other option. Sometimes, though, it's simply a necessity—there's no time or perhaps not enough energy to cook. Whatever the reason, we as a nation have placed part of our health in the hands of restaurant cooks: according to the National Restaurant Association, 54 *billion* meals are eaten in restaurants each year, and on any given day, four out of ten adults dine out.

With so many of us eating out regularly, it's time to start subjecting restaurant fare to the same kind of scrutiny we give our home-cooked meals. It's one thing to dine out on a special night (say, a birthday or an anniversary) and indulge yourself. But if you eat out often, it's important to stop thinking of all restaurant meals as "special" and to start considering them as meals—meals that, because you've made a commitment to your health, should be nutritious, balanced, and reasonably proportioned. It may seem difficult at first, but if each time you step into a restaurant you renew your commitment to the program, you're going to be much more likely to find the inner strength you need to resist the double-cheese pizza.

How to Use This Book

I think you can find something healthy to eat at just about any restaurant, but it can also make a world of difference if you enter an eatery armed with some strategies for navigating the menu or, whenever possible, some advance knowledge about what you can (and can't) count on that particular establishment to offer. More than anything else (except your commitment to stay on track), going in with a plan is your best strategy for staying on the program. That's where this book comes in.

The first section is devoted to some general dining-out tactics that will work just about anywhere. They'll help you sit down in a restaurant—be it an American-style coffee shop, a funky Mexican taco stand, or a swanky French bistro—scan the menu, and zero in on the healthy choices. I also want you to learn to be able to read between the menu lines. If you'd like a vegetarian meal but the restaurant doesn't offer a vegetarian plate, create your own by ordering a bunch of vegetable side dishes. If a restaurant offers fried chicken and grilled steaks, it's possible that it may grill a chicken breast for you if you ask (it obviously has a grill if it's grilling steaks!). Thinking "outside the box" can often net you a meal much healthier than the ones a chef has put on the menu.

The second section of this book is a comprehensive guide to the majority of national and regional chain restaurants in this country. I've looked at menus and pored over nutrition statistics (when available) to find out how each place rates on the health-o-meter as well as to see what its best (and worst) offerings are. Every place, I found, has something to offer, but some places have a greater number of healthy options than others. For that reason, I suggest you use the guide to help you shop around for a restaurant. By browsing through the pages, you can compare and contrast chains before you go, rather than just picking a place and hoping for the best. Why gamble when you can increase the odds that you'll be able to get a healthful meal? You might even keep a copy of this book in the car so that you can consult it when you're on the road rather than settling for the most convenient place.

You can also use this guide to help you determine what you're going to eat before you even get to a restaurant. Meeting a friend at Applebee's or Schlotzsky's Deli? Check out what they have to offer and go knowing that you'll be able to stay on the program once you get there. I find that it really helps steel my own resolve if I do the decision making without a server standing over my shoulder or without the choices my fellow diners have already made to sway me. If you decide what you're going to eat before you go, it will lessen the time you need to look at the menu—and therefore lessen the time the other fattier and more caloric entrees will have to test your determination.

I hope this book will become heavily thumbed as you use it to find the dining spots and different dishes that will help you stay on the program. I think it's important to remember that no single over-the-top restaurant meal will cause you to gain a lot of weight or wipe away all of the healthy eating and exercise that went before it. But eating a large number of unhealthy restaurant meals over time *can* undo a lot of the good you've done, so be vigilant. You now have in your hands all the information you need to make wise choices while still experiencing the pleasures and convenience of dining out (or bringing food in).

For more information about Get With the Program or Bob Greene, log onto www.getwith theprogram.org.

Part I

The Art of Healthful Restaurant Dining

One measure of a successful dining experience is that the patron leaves feeling good about the restaurant. My measure of a successful experience is a little different. I want you to leave a restaurant feeling good about *yourself*. By that I mean that you were able to get a meal that satisfied both your senses and your sense of commitment to leading a healthier life. Ideally, you should never have to leave a restaurant feeling as though you had to compromise your well-being. This becomes much easier if you chose a place that offers quite a few good options.

I'm going to tell you more about how to find restaurants that make it easier to eat healthfully, but first I think it's important to recap just what it is that constitutes good eating. My philosophy is that it takes more than just a good working knowledge of nutrition to change your eating habits for life and lose weight for good. You need to walk before you can run! That's why in the first book in this series, *Get With the Program,* I covered the initial steps that I've found help people get on track to a slimmer, healthier body: making a commitment to yourself, becoming stronger and healthier through exercise, and getting a grip on emotional eating.

The second book, *The Get With the Program! Guide to Good Eating,* is aimed at helping you decipher the glut of nutrition information out there so you can choose good-quality food in reasonable quantities—the key to healthful eating and weight loss.

Now I want you to get a handle on restaurant dining. I hope that at this point, whether you have read the other books or not, you already have a pretty good grasp on the components of a healthy diet. Let's review the basics as they apply to restaurant food.

What Defines a "Good" Restaurant Meal?

The best restaurant meals have the same (or close to the same) healthful qualities your home-prepared meals have. Here are six attributes to keep in mind before you order.

A moderate number of calories. "Moderation" can be an infuriating word. Nutritionists use it all the time, the government advises it, and still nobody really knows what it means. My definition of a moderate-calorie meal is a meal that leaves you neither stuffed nor feeling super-hungry. But it's also important to look at your meals in the larger context of your daily calorie intake.

As you probably already know, to lose weight, you must expend more calories than you consume. It's that simple. But you personally are more complex than a simple equation. You have a certain frame size, your own specific metabolism, a particular amount of activity that you do each day, and your own individual goals. For that reason I can't tell you the exact number of calories you should be taking in. What I *can* tell you is that a good way to judge your calorie needs is to pay attention to your body and its requirements.

First, are you eating enough to satisfy your nutritional needs? You want to get enough carbohydrate, fat, protein, vitamins, minerals, and phytochemicals to keep you healthy. That's of number one importance (and something that many weight-loss plans don't take into account). Second, are you gaining weight, losing weight, or staying the same? That's an obvious indication of whether you're eating too much or too little. Third, how hungry do you feel? If you're trying to maintain your weight, you should eat when you're truly physically hungry and stop before you feel stuffed or are no longer physically hungry. If you want to lose fat, you should stop when you feel as though you'd still like to eat a little at the end of a meal—but just a little. That feeling is your body warning you that it's going to dip into your fat stores, which is exactly what you want to happen.

I think it's healthier to proportion your calories relatively equally throughout the day rather than eating (as many people do) a tiny breakfast, a good-size lunch, and the big traditional American dinner. Ideally, it's best if you can even consume more of your calories in the earlier part of the day; however, no one meal should be overly large—that can trigger an unhealthy insulin surge (more on this in a moment). If you eat a moderately sized breakfast, lunch, and dinner, plus one or two small snacks during the day, you'll be on the right track. (Remember, of course, that if you want to lose weight, the total calories of your meals will need to be lower than the number of calories you burn during the day.)

Over the years, most people have gotten used to the idea of having their largest meal at dinnertime, but there are several reasons not to follow that tradition. You see, each time you eat, your body responds by increasing your metabolism. But your metabolism also has a natural arc to it, which appears to decline as it gets closer to bedtime. By the time you're asleep, it'll have nearly shut down, which may be why the food you eat in the evening doesn't increase your calorie-burning ability as much as the food you eat earlier in the day. Your body, once it's settled into its resting mode, doesn't want to get revved up again.

Another reason it's important to distribute your calories carefully is the fact that eating the majority of your calories at one meal can create an insulin spike, causing your body to store fat. When you take in a high dose of calories—and, in particular, carbohydrate calories—your pancreas gets the message to pump out more insulin than is ideal. Insulin is responsible for moving glucose (blood sugar) out of the bloodstream and into the body's tissues; large amounts of insulin increase the likelihood that the glucose will be stored as fat. An insulin spike caused by a big meal will encourage your body to tuck away more fat—no matter when that oversize meal occurs. If, however, you spread your calories out over many hours, your insulin will stay at a reasonable level and your body will be less likely to hoard fat.

While you should always aim to have a moderate-calorie meal—whether that means ordering sensibly or wrapping up half of a big meal and taking it home—there will be times when you end up eating a restaurant meal higher in calories than you'd like. Just keep things in perspective, it's eating supersize dinners consistently that's going to be detrimental to your health. Just pare down your next meal (or meals) a bit or be a little more active the next day to get back on an even keel. You can even take action immediately after eating. If time allows, grab your dining companion and go for a postmeal walk.

Appropriate portion sizes. It will be a lot easier to keep your calories in check if the meals you order are reasonably proportioned. Here is what a healthy "serving" looks like:

- A serving of rice (and other grains), pasta, or potatoes is equal to ½ cup—which looks like half a tennis ball. A one-serving baked potato can fit in the palm of your hand. (A lot of restaurant baked potatoes are giant-sized!)
- A serving of meat, fish, or poultry weighs 3 to 4 ounces and looks the size of a deck of cards or a computer mouse. (Anything in excess of that, set aside to take home.)
- A serving of cheese is 1 ounce, about the size of your thumb.
- A serving of cooked vegetables is ½ cup, 1 cup for fresh greens. I wouldn't worry about the portion size of vegetables as long as you're eating them without added fats. A serving of fruit is ½ cup—again, half a tennis ball.
- A serving of dairy is 1 cup, the size of a full tennis ball.

A good balance of fat, protein, and carbohydrate. To be healthy, a meal needn't have an ideal percentage of each nutrient—what's important is that you get a good balance of fat, protein, and carbohydrate throughout the day. If one meal is short on protein, for example, you can always make up for it later. But I also think that the *best-case* scenario is to eat a meal that combines the three main nutrients in reasonable proportions. What's reasonable? It's hard to say specifically. Each of us has genetic differences and different levels of activity that influence our metabolic rates and, by extension, our dietary needs.

That said, there are some safe percentages of fat, carbohydrate, and protein that you can start with, then tweak as necessary. I suggest you begin by breaking down your total number of calories in this way: 50 to 55 percent carbohydrates, 25 to 30 percent fat, and 15 to 20 percent protein. See how these proportions work for you—and by that I mean how they make you feel, how much energy they give you, and how well they're helping you accomplish your goal of attaining or maintaining a healthy weight—then adjust and readjust as necessary. In general, the more active you are, the more carbohydrates you can handle.

In regard to an individual meal, consider that fat, protein, and carbohydrate complement one another, which is why the best meal has a combination of all three. Fat and protein, for instance, slow the digestion of carbohydrate; they keep your blood sugar from rising too quickly and causing a corresponding surge in insulin. Having some fat and protein on the plate will also keep you from getting hungry again too quickly, helping to control your appetite and keep you from excess snacking. Fat also makes food more palatable; it tastes good and makes you feel as though you've eaten a "real" meal.

Carbohydrates also have an important place on the plate. For one thing, they generally come with important nutrients, including fiber (more on fiber in a minute), and they also have an effect on how satisfying you find a meal. One of the reasons many people end up going off low-carbohydrate, high-protein diets (and gaining back the weight they lost) is that they miss the taste and texture of carbs.

Just as the calorie count of your restaurant meal may not end up being perfect, its breakdown may not end up being ideal either. But this doesn't have to be a problem; you can balance out your intake on other meals or snacks later.

Reasonable amounts of healthy fats and an absence of unhealthy fats. Contrary to what the whole fat-free boom has led us to believe, fats are an important part of the diet. That is, *healthy* fats are an important part of the diet. The difference between olive oil and margarine is a big one.

A healthy fat is a fat that decreases the risk of heart disease by lowering LDL ("bad") cholesterol and triglyceride levels. Some healthy fats also raise the level of HDL ("good") cholesterol in the blood, helping to keep the arteries free and clear. An unhealthy fat, on the other hand, raises LDL cholesterol and triglyceride levels and can even lower HDL levels.

The healthiest fats are olive and canola oils. Both of these have a large percentage of heart-healthy monounsaturated fatty acids. (Almond, sunflower, avocado and peanut oils, peanut butter, cashews, walnuts, and almonds are all also high in monounsaturates.) Another class of vegetable oils are the polyunsaturated fats. These include corn, soybean, safflower, and fish oils. In addition, omega-3 fatty acids, found in high-fat fish (salmon, tuna, mackerel) and flaxseed, also have a number of health benefits, including reducing the risk of heart disease and possibly other inflammatory conditions.

There are basically two types of unhealthy fats: saturated fats and trans fats. Saturated fats are those found in animal foods such as whole-milk dairy products and red meat. Coconut milk, coconut oil, and palm oil also contain saturated fat. (However, their positive and negative effects on our health are being debated.) Trans fats are generally vegetable oils that have been put through a process called hydrogenation in order to make them solid or semisolid. They're found in most margarines and shortenings and, because they're often used for frying, are abundant in fast foods. They have a long shelf life, so they're also found in a lot of processed foods such as snack crackers and cookies. Researchers now believe that trans fats are even worse for you than saturated fats. There is, for instance, some solid evidence that trans fats raise bad LDL cholesterol and triglyceride levels, while lowering good HDL cholesterol levels. They may also increase the risk of blood clots.

It's often difficult to tell what kind of fats are used to make a restaurant meal, but it doesn't hurt to ask. Many restaurants make a point of using olive and/or canola oil and, if they don't advertise it on the menu already, will be happy to tell you so. Many fast-food restaurants also now list the ingredients, including the fats, on their Web sites, and some even include the exact number of grams of trans and saturated fats found in individual menu items. A few even list the trans fat content of their food, something you will be probably be seeing more of soon. The government has mandated that food manufacturers list trans fat content by 2006, and one can hope that restaurants will follow suit.

Whether or not trans and saturated fat contents are listed on a restaurant's nutritional information page, there are some obvious red flags you can look for. If an entrée is covered with cheese, drowning in a cream sauce or butter, or topped with bacon bits, you can bet it's high in saturated fat. Trans fats are not as easy to detect, but you can ask if a dish is made with margarine and watch out for anything fried.

Occasionally, in the guide to specific restaurants that begins on page 52, you'll see that I recommend ordering a fat-free salad dressing or other fat-free food. This isn't because I think you need to keep your diet fat free. As I've said, reasonable amounts of healthy fats are an important part of the diet. But restaurants generally add fat to food in so many places that I think the more you can do to keep your meal moderately lean, the better. Fats, even good fats, are high in calories, so it's important to keep them in check. Whenever you can get a cook to prepare your food with minimal added fat, do so. Chefs want their food to taste good, so they generally make liberal use of oils and butters unless directed otherwise. A gentle reminder that you're perfectly willing to forgo all that fat will generally help.

Fiber and phytochemicals. Fiber plays a significant role in keeping the body healthy, and it can be a great ally in weight loss. It aids in removing waste products from the body, slows down digestion, and provides volume to help satisfy your hunger. Some of the best sources of fiber are whole grains, but sadly, beyond a few health food and macrobiotic eateries, most restaurants do not serve them. If a restaurant does, take advantage of it: order the whole-grain toast, the brown rice, the oatmeal or All-Bran; whole grains also have other important nutrients besides fiber, such as antioxidants, that may help guard against disease.

If you're at a restaurant that doesn't offer whole grain foods, fruits and vegetables are another good source of fiber. A stir-fry or a fruit salad can help you bulk up your diet, as can ordering several sides of vegetables with your entrée. Getting a liberal amount of fruits and vegetables in your diet will also help you increase your intake of phytochemicals. Phytochemicals are compounds made by plants that have a beneficial effect on the body. Scientists are only beginning to scratch the surface of the usefulness of these compounds, but they do know that the more phytochemical-rich fruits and vegetables we get in our diets, the lower our risk of disease. A general rule of thumb is that the more brightly colored the fruit or vegetable, the more phytochemicals it contains, so choose a colorful meal.

Lean protein. We all need protein. It provides the basis for building, maintaining, and repairing body tissues—something, especially as an active person, you cannot do without. Protein also helps you burn calories, and in fact it precipitates a bigger thermic effect—a surge in calorie burning triggered by eating—than any other nutrient. You may have been led to believe that you need to eat heaps of protein, but that isn't the case. If you eat protein to the exclusion of carbohydrates and fat, your body will break down your muscles for energy, limiting the amount of calories you burn (muscle requires a lot of energy to maintain, and the more you have of it, the more calories you burn, even at rest).

Making 15 to 20 percent of your total calories protein foods is adequate, but it's also critical to make sure that you choose the *right* protein foods. Animal sources of protein tend to go hand in hand with saturated fat, but lean sources have only minimal amounts. I'm not saying you shouldn't eat red meat, but I think you'll find that restaurants tend to use fattier cuts (they're more tender), so you're better off sticking to fish and other seafood, egg whites (a few egg yolks a week are okay if you do not have elevated cholesterol), white-meat poultry, and lean cuts of pork. If you do order red meat, ask for the dishes that use leaner cuts, such as sirloin and round, and trim any obvious fat off yourself.

You can also, of course, get protein through nonanimal sources, such as nuts, seeds, legumes, dairy products, and soy products such as tofu. If a restaurant serves soy patties (for example, Boca Burgers) or tofu, take advantage of them. Just be certain you know how they're prepared. Tofu, especially at Asian restaurants, is often served fried. Whole-milk dairy products, of course, also contain a lot of fat (and it's saturated fat), so stick with nonfat or low-fat options.

Minimally processed ingredients. In an ideal world, every dish you order at a restaurant would be made from fresh food, with no preservatives, chemicals, or ridiculous amounts of added sugars and salt. In the real world, restaurants often use processed products—higher-end places less so, but less expensive restaurants usually depend on them to keep their prices down. Keep a watchful eye. Whenever possible, order dishes made "fresh" on the premises, such as salads, homemade soups, and vegetable sides.

Drinks without added sugar or chemicals. One thing that every restaurant has is water, your top drink choice. Those of you who have read my previous books know that I am a fierce advocate of drinking lots of water throughout the day—a minimum of six eight-ounce glasses a day and preferably more like nine. Here's why: Being dehydrated diminishes the body's ability to perform virtually every physiological function, including fat metabolism. Dehydration also makes your body go in search of water, but somewhere along the way it gets interpreted as hunger—a phenomenon I call "artificial hunger"—and causes you to end up eating more than you should. Dehydration also causes the digestive system to work at a diminished capacity, potentially preventing you from getting the nutrients you need and triggering unnecessary eating to make up for the shortfall.

So water is what you should drink. If you find water just too boring, consider the new flavored vitamin waters being served at some places. They have a touch of flavor and very few calories. What shouldn't you drink? Avoid sodas, which are really just sugar, water, and artificial flavor, and diet sodas, which are water and chemicals with little redeeming nutritional value. Juices—at least some juices—do offer many vitamins, but they are also highly caloric, so I suggest you limit your intake or order your juice cut in half with club soda (it will also halve the calories).

Chances are, you're going to eat more calories when dining out than you would at home; ordering a drink with a substantial number of calories will just bump up the number even more. And those beverage calories can really add up. For example, one 20-ounce soda has about 250 calories. If you get two refills, you've consumed 750 calories of nutrient-free soda, more calories than you probably want to consume for your entire meal! For similar calorie-related reasons (and others), alcohol is another drink I recommend you limit; I'll talk a little more about that in a later section.

The danger of ordering coffee at a restaurant is that it's often a bottomless cup—get assigned a friendly waitress, and before you know it you've downed five cups! And if you take your coffee with cream and sugar, it won't only be excess caffeine you're getting. Many people don't even register the calories they get from adding cream (which also has saturated fat), most artificial creamers, and sugar to their coffee. Yet they can add up to quite a bit if you're drinking more than one cup.

If you're a regular coffee drinker, I recommend switching to decaf as often as possible, if not entirely. Likewise with tea. Most restaurants offer decaffeinated coffee, and many also offer herb or decaffeinated black teas. Consider ordering green tea. Although it has some caffeine, it also has phytochemicals, which researchers have found may protect against many diseases, including cancer. If you prefer iced tea but your dining spot doesn't offer any of the healthier variations, order hot herbal or green tea and a big cup of ice and make your own.

Before I go on, I just want to reiterate that it's not important that every meal you eat be perfect. You may find yourself in a restaurant where you just can't seem to find anything on the program to eat. Or you may find yourself in a restaurant on a day when you're feeling vulnerable or in the mood to indulge—there are healthy things on the menu, but you just decide not to order them. Either way, you're going to be fine. It takes 3,500 calories to gain a pound, and that's quite a bit more than one splurge.

What matters most is consistency. If you eat healthfully 90 percent of the time, those rare restaurant sprees aren't going to harm you. Just don't get caught up in thinking that you've blown it, so why not blow it some more? Enjoy yourself and recommit to the program at the next meal.

Restaurant Reconnaissance: Picking the Right Place Is Half the Battle

Convenience is often the reason people give for choosing a particular restaurant. Force of habit is another. But if those reasons have you tethered to a spot that doesn't really suit your needs, I hope you'll shake up your routine and find a better place (or places). The sure way to get a healthy meal when dining out is to go to a restaurant that pays attention to its customers' needs. The best places either have plenty of sensible choices on the menu or welcome special orders.

The guide at the back of this book will help you get a feel for which chains fit that criteria (and which don't), but to find out what independent eateries can offer you, you're going to have to do a little legwork. Here are the criteria you should use to find a "good" restaurant.

Does it offer several healthy entrées? Many restaurants position themselves as "splurgeterias"—places where people are *supposed* to indulge. When that's the case, they usually don't bother putting anything low in fat and calories on the menu—and, of course, that's their prerogative. *Your* prerogative is to dine somewhere else. To my mind, the best type of restaurant is one that has not just one or two but many healthy options on the menu. Don't get me wrong—I'll take one or two; however, limited options can get boring. You're more likely to stray into the indulgent area of the menu if the nutritious side dishes are restricted to, say, one big salad with fat-free dressing or an egg-white omelet. So whenever possible, choose a restaurant that has varied low and moderate calorie choices.

Will they prepare food "your way"? The two words I hate to see on a restaurant menu are *"No substitutions."* I can understand why some fast-food restaurants live by that credo since it helps them get food out fast, as the label implies (although some of them don't get food out as fast as they'd have you believe). But even some fast-food joints are open to fulfilling special requests, and it seems to me that a place that makes food to order should be able to accommodate customers' (reasonable) demands. That said, many places are very obliging, and this is particularly true if you're a regular customer.

If it doesn't have a particularly healthy menu, does it at least have enough of a selection to allow you to cobble together a healthy meal? As I mentioned, there are restaurants that are meant for splurging and restaurants that stubbornly resist substitutions and other requests. Sometimes, if the menu is large enough, you can work around these limitations. It might be just a matter of ordering two first-course appetizers (such as soup and salad) instead of a first course and an oversized entrée. Perhaps you might order from the list of side dishes (a baked potato and a side of spinach or mixed vegetables). Such a meal might not always be perfect, but it's a good way to stay on the program in a pinch, and you can always make up for what you might be missing (in the case of the above examples, protein) at your next meal.

Now that I've given you my definition of the best kinds of restaurants, you'll need to go out and identify them. Say, for instance, there are several cafés and bistros near your workplace. Collect menus from all of them. See which of them have the most health-conscious offerings, then make it a point to patronize those restaurants. Knowing the menus of several restaurants will also help you steer colleagues and other business associates to the places that you know serve healthful dishes, rather than letting them steer you to places where you'll have a hard time finding anything you want to eat. The same goes for restaurants near your house. Do the research; you may find that some of them have better options than you expected.

Do some reconnaissance before you travel as well. This may be as simple as looking through guidebooks to find restaurants with healthy selections or, if necessary, making a few phone calls. If you'll be staying at a hotel with a concierge, phone ahead and ask for suggestions. He or she probably already knows a few places. The concierge or the restaurant you're interested in may even be able to fax you a menu at home before you leave. Or look on the Web; you may find everything there that you need to know.

If you're going on a road trip, the smartest thing you can do is pack your own food. But if that's not practical, find out what restaurants will be on the route you're traveling. If you know that, for instance, you can always find something healthy at Denny's, go to the Denny's Web site and check its restaurant locator to see if there's a branch on your travel route, then plan your stops accordingly. This might sound a little obsessive, but there is nothing worse than being stuck on the road and forced to eat at a place where the healthy pickings are slim. A little foresight can make a big difference.

Finally, become a menu collector. I have a special drawer at home devoted to a stash of menus from restaurants in my area. This not only helps me know what will be in store for me before I go but also gives me a chance to think about what I'm going to order. I find that it's often easier to make healthy choices if you don't have the pressure of the waitperson standing over you while you try to decide. Going in with your mind already made up about what you're going to have can also help you resist the kind of why-not-join-the-gang pressure when everyone else starts ordering fried calamari and cheese-drenched nachos.

Basic Strategies for Staying on the Program

To some extent, when you dine out you're always going to be somewhat at the mercy of the restaurants you go to. You *can,* though, can take certain aspects of restaurant dining into your own hands. Here are some tips.

- *Stand your ground when it comes to choosing a restaurant.*

  Sometimes it's friends, sometimes it's family, sometimes it's business colleagues—there are many people who may try to pressure you into eating at a place that you know is going to make it difficult for you to find something healthful to eat. If you can't persuade your dining partners to go to your top choice, at least find a compromise. Keep in mind, too, that there are other places to have business meetings and/or socialize beside restaurants. Meet for tea or a drink at a place where you can order something nonalcoholic. Go to the movies and out to a coffeehouse afterwards, rather than to the movies and dinner. In the summer suggest a picnic so that you can bring the food you want to eat, or consider entertaining at home so that you can make a healthy meal.

- *Snack a little before you go out.*

  This is an old trick, but it works—and not just for keeping your ordering under control at restaurants. It's also a great technique for ensuring that you don't overeat (or overdrink) at parties. The idea is this: When you arrive at a restaurant (or an event with food) feeling famished, you are going to want to attack the first plate of food you see. At a restaurant, that's usually the breadbasket, at a party the tray of appetizers. When you're hungry, your rumbling stomach is going to overrule your rational mind when it comes to ordering, leading you to order the steak with bleu cheese sauce; satiety will keep you cool, calm, and collected enough to order the grilled fish.

- *Avoid the bar.*

  I don't believe that everyone needs to be a teetotaler to stay on the program. But I do believe that you're better off being an occasional drinker. Some wines and spirits contain antioxidants, but for the most part, alcohol calories are empty calories that you don't need. They offer you no fiber, vitamins, or minerals. If you're so inclined, have a drink or a glass of wine once in a while for pleasure, but don't make alcohol a regular part of your day.

Restaurants like to get you into the bar whenever possible. They make a lot of money off alcohol (even more than they make off food), so it's not surprising that the hostess will try to steer you to the bar while you wait for your table. If you do end up at the bar and you feel compelled to order something, ask for a juice spritzer (juice cut with carbonated water) or mineral water.

- *Decline wine and other alcoholic drinks at the table.*

  As soon as you get to the table, your server will undoubtedly come around pushing more alcohol (servers always seem disappointed if you don't order wine). Resist the pressure. These days, servers in finer restaurants also generally try to push bottled mineral water. Water, is always good in my book, and if ordering a bottle will get you to drink more of it during your meal (water from the tap in some municipalities tastes awful), go for it. Sometimes just the idea that you've paid for it will induce you to drink it! Yes, restaurants tend to overcharge for mineral water, but you'll be much better off if you spend your money on water rather than on alcohol or soda.

- *Ask your server not to bring the bread basket (or chips if you're in a Mexican restaurant).*

  Even if you've vowed to have just a single piece of bread, you may find it hard to resist going for more, especially if you have to wait a long time for your meal. It's easier not to have the bread on the table. If your dining companions want bread, you can ask them to keep the basket away from your side of the table. You can also take a portion of bread or chips and then ask the server to remove the basket.

• *Make your server your ally.*

Your waiter or waitress is your conduit to the kitchen and key to getting what you want. Thus, the better your communication with your server, the better your meal will be. Learn and use your server's first name. Make eye contact, explain what you want, ask questions. If you're a regular at a restaurant and know you can count on a particular server to be receptive to your needs, request to be put in his or her section. You want to have the person who'll make sure your salad dressing comes on the side and that your toast is dry, not slathered in butter.

• *Look at the ingredients, not just the dishes listed on a menu.*

What you see on the menu is not all that you can get. If, for instance, a restaurant offers omelettes, it can probably also make you an egg-white omelette. If pasta with broccoli is an entrée, it can probably also bring you a side of broccoli with your chicken. You'll find that some menus are written in stone, but most restaurants will allow you some leeway—they want you to leave happy. It certainly doesn't hurt to ask. If they say no, just be gracious— and then cross that restaurant off your list of accommodating places.

• *Order small portions.*

This might seem like a tall order, given the fact that the portion sizes in restaurants these days border on the obscene. You can often get around this by splitting a meal with your dining partner or having your server wrap up half of your meal so you can take it home. Sometimes restaurants charge a split fee, which I admit is annoying. But you'll be doing yourself a favor if you just pony up the modest fee. (Some places don't actually make you pay it.) You'll end up with a healthier meal and you'll save money.

Another way to get around the big-portion dilemma is to order appetizers as your entrée: soup or salad and an appetizer or two appetizers and one entrée split between two people. If your dining companion isn't willing to share, many finer restaurants will also shave entrées down to smaller, appetizer proportions if you ask.

• *Pass on the buffet.*

America, I know, loves buffets. Economically, I have to agree that they're a bargain, a lot of food for a moderate amount of money. But what are you really getting? The food is never as hot or as good as food that's been made to order. Other people (perhaps even sniffling and sneezing people) have been poking at the buffet before you, and, I don't know about you, but standing in line for food makes me feel a little like cattle. Plus a buffet isn't really conducive to enjoying the company you're with. As soon as you sit down, your dining companion is up and back for seconds. It's like musical chairs!

The worst thing about buffets is that they're an invitation to overeat. It's hard not to want to sample everything and thus hard not to end up taking in more calories than you should, even if your portions are small. Salad bars are better than full buffets since the choices are limited, though you still need to be careful about piling your plate too high with calorie-heavy "add-ins" and drowning it all in high-fat dressing. If you do find yourself at a buffet, try this strategy: eat only the things that you really, really love and forgo things that you can get elsewhere or make at home. Better yet, save the buffets for at-home potlucks with family and friends. At least then you can add some healthy dishes of your own to the table—and you won't feel as though you need to eat "your money's worth."

- *Beware of hidden calories.*

Not all dishes that sound healthy actually are. As I surveyed restaurant menus for this book, I found that many nutritious-sounding dishes, such as some of the chicken salads, actually had more saturated fat and/or calories than the foods that you'd expect to be worse (such as simple hamburgers). Find out how something is made before you order it. For instance, is the chicken in the chicken sandwich breaded and fried or grilled without the skin? Does a salad have cheese and fried noodles or chips mixed in? Does the turkey come swimming in gravy? Get the facts before you order.

- *Be smart when it comes to salads.*

Salads often sound healthy but in reality may not be. What's more, a healthy salad can be made considerably less healthy just by the dressing you choose to put on it. Many places now offer reduced-fat and low-calorie dressings, which can really help improve the quality of your salad. But when they don't, order your dressings on the side and rather than pouring the dressing on your salad, dip your fork into it, then take a bite of salad. Very little dressing sticks to the tines of the fork, but you'll get some of its flavor with each bite. You can also use a little bit of oil and vinegar or lemon juice instead of prepared dressing.

- *Don't let "eating like a bird" jokes bother you.*

For some reason best left to psychologists to explain, people don't like to see others eating healthfully when they are eating poorly. I guess it has something to do with guilt. It's not your job to make other people feel comfortable with their decisions to overindulge. Your decision to make healthful changes in your life was made on behalf of yourself, not anyone else. Keep that in mind, and I think you'll find it much easier to resist the urgings of friends and family to overeat.

• *Save dessert for later.*

One little trick I play on myself is that instead of ordering dessert at the restaurant, I suggest to my dinner companions that we go somewhere else. Often by the time we drive or walk to the next place, I realize I'm not even hungry anymore and I end up skipping dessert entirely. When you order dessert immediately after dinner, you haven't yet had the chance to get up and see how your body feels. And if you're really still hungry for dessert? Hopefully you've steered your group to a place that serves healthy dessert choices.

What to Eat Where

Although there are many principles for dining out that go for just about any type of restaurant—avoid megaportions, fried foods, butter and full-fat dairy products, cheese, fatty meats, sugary desserts, greasy salad dressings—each type of restaurant requires some specific tactics. Here are some tips that will help you order well no matter where you are.

American Diner/Coffee Shop Food

Though no two places are exactly alike, most coffee shops and diners have the same types of items on their menus. Here are some good (and bad) choices for every meal:

Breakfast: Expect to see an array of egg dishes, pancakes, waffles, and French toast. These hearty breakfasts can really drag you down throughout the day and often come with a lot of saturated fat and cholesterol, especially if they include bacon, sausage, or other breakfast meats. Stick with simple egg dishes: two poached eggs and some whole-wheat toast (avoid the biscuits and have tomatoes or fruit instead of potatoes), for example, or an egg-white omelette stuffed with veggies. I often see

Egg Beaters on the menu, and these are a good option, too. Whole-grain cold cereal or oatmeal, with fruit and either skim or low-fat milk, are all wise choices. Granola can also be a healthy selection, but only if it's low-fat granola. Otherwise it will probably have just as many calories as the French toast!

Lunch: You can't go wrong with a grilled chicken or turkey sandwich on whole-wheat bread, slathered with mustard and topped with lettuce and tomato. A salad can also be a good lunch, but you really have to read the menu closely to see what the ingredients are. It seems that no one likes to make the plain old vegetable-heavy salads anymore; these days, they're almost always junked up with cheese, fatty meats, or crispy noodles. The good news is that you can almost always get the restaurant to hold all the extras and serve you a nice big garden salad—all the better if it has a reduced-fat dressing on hand. Soups are another great lunch option; just stay away from the creamy ones. A grilled chicken sandwich should be picked over the traditional hamburger.

Dinner: Start out with salad or soup—or combine the two to make a complete dinner. It's usually possible to get a grilled or roasted chicken breast; that's always a good pick. Fish is sometimes on the menu, too, though I'd ask if it's fresh before ordering. It won't be any less healthy if it's frozen, but it may not taste so great. Roast turkey and even pot roast are other reasonable options, though in each case you'll need to forgo the gravy, which can drive up the fat and calorie counts considerably. Beware of sides such as stuffing; ask for additional vegetables. As to what *not* to have for dinner, stay away from the fried shrimp, country-fried steak, and pork chops.

Chinese

Here's the good news about Chinese food: These days many places have a health-conscious section (or at the very least an entrée or two) on the menu with dishes that are steamed, made without oil and even without soy sauce. If the thought of Chinese food without sauce leaves you cold, you can order one of the steamed dishes; ask for sauce on the side, and dab it on judiciously. Some Chinese restaurants also prepare steamed fish dishes that come in a light ginger/soy sauce or some variation thereof. These sauces are generally low in fat and make the fish an excellent choice even with the sauce already on.

The bad news about Chinese food is that dishes that sound relatively light, such as chicken and broccoli, can actually be quite caloric because of all the oil used in stir-frying. Skip anything deep-fried, such as sesame or lemon chicken, or breaded, such as orange beef. Forget the egg rolls and go for an appetizer such as egg drop, wonton, or hot and sour soup, or just a simple vegetable soup if they have it. Choose steamed dumplings over fried ones.

Choose entrées that use lean forms of protein, such as white-meat chicken without the skin, fish, shrimp, scallops, or lobster. Something like sliced chicken with mixed vegetables, Szechuan shrimp, or shrimp with asparagus is a good choice. Offerings may vary from one restaurant to the next, but these common selections will give you an idea of the *type* of dish to order, if not the exact dish. Tofu can be a healthy option, but only if it's not fried, so check before ordering. Nuts add healthy fat and protein to a dish but also add calories, so keep that in mind when making your selections. It doesn't hurt to ask if the cook can go easy on the oil. Restaurants often make dishes to order.

One of the pluses of Chinese food is that most dishes include lots of vegetables, and there are often lots of vegetarian options, such as Buddha's Feast. Eggplant is the one vegetable dish I'd advise against, since it soaks up oil like a sponge. At some Chinese restaurants, you can now get brown rice to accompany your meal, a great option. If it's not available, plain white rice is preferable to fried rice and to noodle dishes such as lo mein and chow mein. Go ahead and have the fortune cookie at meal's end: it's only about 30 calories.

French

French food has always been infamous for its high butter and cream content, but I'm happy to say that the food at many French restaurants has lightened up. Nowadays you will see many dishes made with olive oil instead of butter, and sauces are often made with puréed vegetables instead of cream. Also, the portions at French restaurants tend to be smaller than at other restaurants.

When you're having a meal at a French restaurant, I recommend that you start with something light, such as a simple green or vegetable salad. Soup can also be an option if it's a consommé or onion soup without cheese on top. Stay away from the vichyssoise and lobster bisque, both of which are traditionally made with cream. Other appetizers to resist: escargot (swimming in butter) and foie gras. Many French bistros offer mussels, which are not a bad choice; however, ask if they're made with butter before ordering. If they are, reconsider or try to resist the urge to mop up the mussels' brine with bread—that's where the majority of the butter will land.

You can almost always order a fish entrée at a French restaurant. Usually the chef will be willing to grill or broil it for you, or at least sauté it in olive oil instead of butter. Be sure to ask to have any sauce on the side. Many French places serve light fish such as sole and sand dabs, which are a good choice, though you'll probably be able to order salmon and tuna, too. At a bistro, roast chicken is a staple and a good choice; you can discreetly remove the skin before you eat it. You can even enjoy the coq au vin, chicken in wine, if you don't eat the bacon the dish is seasoned with. Forgo the pommes frites (French fries), the usual accompaniment, and ask for vegetable sides instead. Chicken pot-au-feu—chicken with vegetables in a pot— is another relatively healthy choice.

Among the things to avoid are medallions of beef or filet mignon topped with Bearnaise sauce, any kind of mousse (from crab to chocolate), and creamed spinach.

Indian

There's something in almost every Indian dish that is definitely not on the program: ghee, a clarified form of butter that's integral to Indian cooking. For that reason, when eating Indian food, it's important to really watch your portion sizes or the calories (and saturated fat) will add up.

Skip the appetizers here, especially the samosas and pakoras, which are deep-fried. Hands down, the best thing you can order at an Indian restaurant is the tandoori-style dishes. Most places cook everything from chicken, shrimp, fish, and lamb in tandoori fashion. Another reasonable dish is chicken tikka, boneless breast marinated in yogurt and spices, then either grilled tandoori-style or served in a tomato sauce.

Curries, vindaloo, saag, masala, and paneer (with cheese) are all different cooking styles that are used with vegetables, seafood, poultry, and meat. How caloric they are varies from place to place, depending on the amount of ghee used, so enjoy them sparingly. You can reduce their dietary impact by choosing the leanest version—shrimp, for instance, instead of lamb. Fresh breads are another staple of Indian cuisine. Keep your bread consumption under control. Chapati, a whole-wheat bread, is your best choice.

Italian

Italian food is consistently rated one of the most popular ethnic foods in the United States. It can also be one of the most dangerous to your weight loss efforts if you don't order wisely.

Where should you begin? Soup. Most Italian restaurants serve a minestrone or *pasta e fagioli* (pasta and bean soup), either of which will give you a healthy start. Simple salads are okay too, but not the cheese-laden Caesar or greens topped with slices of provolone or Parmesan; ask to have your dressing on the side. A vegetable antipasto might seem like a good choice, but the vegetables have usually been marinated in oil, so stick to simple soups and salads.

The typical American Italian restaurant serves enough pasta in one entrée for two people, so consider splitting an entrée! When you think of Italian food you might consider skipping the pasta and going right to the "secondi" section, which is usually where you'll find the fish, chicken, and meats. Your best bet here is whatever is cooked simply: a roasted fish, a sautéed breast of chicken or veal cutlet, even a grilled piece of pork tenderloin. What you don't want are any of the breaded and fried entrées, the whopping T-bones or veal chops, or the dishes smothered in creamy sauces or cheese. Avoid anything called "parmigiana." If you feel you *can't* resist the pasta, have a simple version with tomato sauce (or red clam sauce) as a side dish. And consider that choice as your starch—in other words, forgo the bread. Or have a piece of bread and forgo the pasta.

Although it's really almost as American as apple pie, let's also talk about pizza. One small slice of pizza and sometimes even two will probably not throw you off your program. But three or four pieces will. If you know you're going to have pizza, try to cut back elsewhere that day, particularly on saturated fat, since the pizza's cheese will send your saturated fat count over the top.

When you eat pizza, I encourage you to stick to the basics: thin crust with cheese and some vegetables (but *not* eggplant) on top (extras such as pepperoni and sausage can really ratchet up the calories and saturated-fat count). If you frequent a pizzeria that makes pies to order, you can even ask it to cut the amount of cheese in half. What you need to watch out for is the nutrition nightmares, like pizzas that have not only cheese on top but also a cheese-stuffed crust. Then, of course, there's the old-fashioned Chicago-style deep-dish pizza. A deep-dish cheese slice can have 480 calories or more, while a thin-crust cheese slice has about 280 calories.

Japanese

You shouldn't have any trouble finding something healthy to eat at a Japanese restaurant—Japanese cuisine is one of the leanest around.

Still, there are a few things you'll need to watch out for. One is sodium, if you're prone to dousing your Japanese food with soy sauce, as so many people are. Many places now place low-sodium soy sauce on the table next to the regular stuff, which will help you cut back. Also consider asking for some rice wine vinegar to flavor your food. It has a wonderful mild nutty flavor, and you can either use it by itself or combine it with soy sauce to give any dish a little zip.

The best way to start your meal at a Japanese restaurant is with miso soup or a green salad (the dressing served with it is usually fairly light, but ask for it on the side nonetheless). Other healthy appetizers are yakitori, skewered and grilled chicken, and edamame (boiled soybeans). Pass on the gyoza, fried dumplings, and tempura, which is vegetables and/or meat, poultry, or fish dipped into a batter and fried.

Sushi (raw fish with rice) and sashimi (raw fish without the rice) are very lean entrées. Teriyaki dishes are also good choices, as are teppan yaki (stir-fries) and sukiyaki (chicken in sauce). Avoid katsu dishes, which are breaded and fried. Many places now serve Japanese noodle dishes with udon or soba noodles. These are generally lean and healthy dishes, but watch the portion sizes, as they often come in huge bowls.

Mexican

There are a few obvious foods to avoid at Mexican restaurants, so let's get those out of the way first. Chips and nachos, of course, but also chimichangas, taquitos, and chiles rellenos, all of which are deep-fried. Quesadillas are often supercheesy, and enchiladas are usually covered with cheese, so avoid them as well. Burritos, while essentially filled with good ingredients (rice, beans, salsa and sometimes chicken), can often be so big that they contain two meals' worth of calories. If the burritos at your local taqueria are supersize, get someone to split one with you or take half home. If they're reasonable in size, a bean, rice, and salsa burrito (hold the cheese!) is a good choice.

Mexican food uses healthful ingredients, but it's often cooked with a lot of fat, including lard. So you have to be selective. For instance, you might wonder how bad a tamale—little packages of cornmeal flavored with vegetables or meat—could be. Unfortunately, it takes a lot of fat to give tamales their smooth texture. A taco salad sounds like a nutritious option; it is, after all, a salad. But if you go to Taco Bell it's also 790 calories! Even if you forgo eating the deep-fried shell, it's 420 calories, more than you might have bargained for.

At more upscale places, the tostadas (a Mexican salad atop a fried tortilla) can also be deceiving. They often include beans that are refried in lard, sour cream, and guacamole. It all adds up to quite a calorie fest. That said, it's possible to order a tostada and do right by yourself. Just ask for the chef to hold the sour cream and guacamole and don't eat the shell. Use the salsa on the table (which usually doesn't contain any fat) as dressing. I, in fact, put salsa on everything—the flavor is so intense that you won't miss the cheese or any other fatty extras. Of course, salsa is usually served with chips, which you don't want to eat. However, some restaurants will bring you carrots and other vegetables for dipping or serve pickled vegetables and radishes as a substitute for chips.

Many places offer plain black and pinto beans that haven't been refried and are cooked without oil. If you can get those, a bowl of beans with a side of rice is a great Mexican meal. Some restaurants and fast-food eateries are now also serving lighter variations on traditional dishes, but if your local place doesn't, try ordering from the à la carte side of the menu. Besides rice and beans, you can often order single tacos and enchiladas (ask them to hold the cheese). In general, tacos, hard or soft, aren't very fattening, especially if you get a chicken or fish taco (just make sure the fish hasn't been deep-fried).

Fajitas are another good choice: they are essentially fish, shrimp, chicken, or lean meats grilled with vegetables. Fajitas are often served with extras and tortillas on the side. Your best bet is to skip them both, though if you feel the need to have a tortilla, ask for corn rather than flour—it will be lower in calories and a little higher in fiber.

Thai

Thai cooks use a lot of garlic, chilies, onions, and lemon grass to flavor food, so much Thai food is wonderfully flavored without being smothened in sauce. However, it also has some of the same dietary pitfalls as Chinese food: lots of fat and calories slipped into savory sauces and mixed dishes. Get off on the right foot here by ordering reasonable appetizers. Chicken satay, which is generally grilled white meat on a skewer, is a smart start, as are light broth soups such as vegetable wonton and tom yum kai, a spicy soup with vegetables. (Don't mistake it for tom kha kai, which contains coconut milk and a lot more calories.) Thai restaurants usually serve salads, which are also a good choice; however, go easy on the dressing, which is typically made from peanuts.

Noodle dishes—particularly Pad Thai—are a big draw. However, I suggest that if you're going to order one, you share it and keep your portion small. Choose lean forms of protein, such as white-meat chicken without the skin, fish, shrimp, or scallops, as well as mixed vegetable dishes. It's probably best to pass on the curries—it's hard to know just how much fat is in them—and stick to dishes stir-fried with lighter sauces or just garlic and chilies.

Ask your server what the lightest dishes are, then follow his or her advice.

Part II

THE GUIDE

This guide to eating at chain restaurants grew out of my own desire to know where I could find a healthy meal, as well as to fill a void in the information already out there. Although you can find lots of guides to the restaurants in a city, few (if any) of them tell you if you'll be able to get a meal that's rich in nutrients and low in calories. Since I'm moving around the country a lot, I need to know not just who's the hottest chef in a town I'm visiting but where I can grab a quick lunch that won't drag me down the rest of the day. And even when I'm at home, I want to know which places in my area cater to people who care about their health.

I hope that having this information on hand will help you, too. But before you read on, I want to tell you a little bit about how I assembled the information and what I think is the best approach to using it.

As you might expect, I didn't go to every branch of every chain restaurant in the country. What I did instead was to peruse the menus from each chain, talk to people at the various branches of the restaurants, and study the nutritional information of their food whenever available. This gave me a good sense of not only the restaurants' receptiveness to the needs of health-conscious eaters but also what specifically is on their menus that fits in with the program.

Nonetheless, I want to add a few caveats. First, you should know that while the menus at chain restaurants are fairly standard, they can vary regionally and sometimes even within the same town. So there may be something the guide says is offered at a certain restaurant, but you can't find it on your menu. Hopefully, the restaurant will have other healthy choices so that you won't be left out in the cold.

Also, keep in mind that restaurants change their menus. I've tried to be as up to date as possible and even tried to get a jump on things by asking companies if they expected to put any new and healthy offerings on their menus in the near future. What I learned is that restaurants are very proprietary (and understandably so—it's a very competitive business) and are usually reluctant to discuss what they've got in the works. So it's possible that you may even find some great dishes being offered that aren't listed here. On the flip side, you may also find that some of the dishes listed here have been discontinued. I think that the more we show restaurants that we're willing to order healthy dishes, the more likely they are to keep them on the menu.

My hope is that you'll find the information in this guide indispensable and that you'll keep it close at hand so that you can choose restaurants wisely whenever you're eating out. You may want to keep a copy in your car's glove compartment or your travel bag. You can also check out the Web sites of the restaurants you plan to visit. Most chains (and even many restaurants that are not part of a chain) have Web sites that have extensive nutrition information, more than is provided here. Taking a look at it can only help make you an even better informed restaurant consumer.

As you read through the guide, I also hope it will give you a sense of what to order at *any* restaurant, whether it's listed here or not. By listing the good dishes (what I call "Top Picks") as well as the bad (called "Not on the Program") at each restaurant, my goal is to provide specific recommendations as well as to give you a general sense of intelligent ordering. You may not have, say, an Olive Garden near you, but if you live close to an Italian restaurant that serves similar dishes, use the Olive Garden's recommendations to help guide your selections.

Here are some other specifics that will help you use this guide:

• *Calorie counts:* You'll notice that sometimes calorie counts are provided, sometimes not. That's because only some restaurants make this information available. When it is available, I've passed it on to you so that you can get a good idea of how many of your total daily calories a restaurant meal will provide. I also wanted you to be able to compare dishes at one restaurant to one another as well as to dishes at other establishments. Each calorie count is for one serving (as dished out by the restaurant).

You may notice that the calorie counts on some "Top Picks" are higher than others. This is simply because the lowest-calorie offerings at some places are considerably more caloric than the lowest-calorie offerings at other places. When you see a dish that seems a little high in calories, it's because it's the best the restaurant has to offer. Remember that one meal does not a whole day make. If you prefer to eat a higher-calorie meal when dining out, just cut back elsewhere during the day.

Although I frequently point out when a dish is very fatty—or is *low* in saturated and total fat—I haven't included fat counts. Be assured, though, that I did take fat into consideration when recommending specific dishes. On occasion I even opted *not* to recommend certain dishes that were relatively low in calories because they were too high in saturated or trans fat. When contemplating a dish, I also considered whether it was filled with "bad" (i.e., refined) carbohydrates and whether it was a good source of fiber, whole grains, fruits, and vegetables.

• What's "Not on the Program": If I were to include all the dishes that I *don't* recommend under the heading "Not on the Program" the lists would take up volumes. But rather than just instructing you to avoid everything else that's not a top pick, I decided to list a few dishes that were particularly egregious. Some dishes were so outrageously oversized and high in calories that I included them just so you can see what you're up against! Even if restaurants are getting better at providing healthy options, there are still a lot of over-the-top dishes to be had. I also included dishes with names that make them sound healthy but surprisingly are not.

• *Some things go without saying:* Rather than tell you again and again not to go for certain types of food, I'd prefer that you just remember that certain restaurant-prepared foods (and beverages) are off limits when you're trying to stick to the program. They are: fried foods, including French fries, onion rings, tortilla chips, wonton noodles; dishes smothered in cheese; creamy soups; creamy sauces; mayonnaise-based condiments; starchy breakfast foods such as pancakes, waffles, and French toast; doughnuts and pastries (especially those now-ubiquitous cinnamon buns); milk shakes; sodas (remember, lots of places serve unsweetened iced tea, and they *all* have water). I also hardly ever comment on appetizers because at many places they are little more than platters of grease (the usual suspects, such as fried mozzarella sticks, buffalo wings, nachos, and fried dumplings). Throughout the guide I often recommend that, when available, you choose reduced-fat and fat-free salad dressings, although it's not an absolute must. But when you do use regular salad dressing, order it on the side and use it very sparingly.

I have chosen not to include most doughnut shops, cinnamon bun shops, ice cream shops, and other purveyors of sweets in this guide. That's because they rarely serve anything that might be considered a "Top Pick," plus I think you know that when you enter one of these places you're heading for trouble. Remember your commitment to yourself, and it will likely be easier for you to pass them by.

Eating out healthfully may be getting easier, but it still requires stick-to-itiveness. Although the dining advice given here will certainly help you, in the end it's your strong desire to change your life for the better that's going to do the trick. But you've already started the ball rolling just by looking to this book to help you bone up on restaurant facts. Now go out there and eat well!

★ = Best Bet: A restaurant with many healthy choices

A&W ALL AMERICAN RESTAURANTS

www.awrestaurants.com

A&W restaurants have been around for a long time, and their menu remains fairly small. You probably won't find any foods aimed at the health-conscious here, but you can still dine at A&W without going off the program if you order wisely. That means keeping it simple, leaving off fatty sauces, and—need I say it?—resisting the fries and onion rings.

Top Picks

Sandwiches:

- Grilled Chicken—Hold the sauce.
- Hamburger—The chicken is a leaner choice, but if you feel compelled to have meat, this is your best choice. Again, hold the sauce. A&W doesn't provide nutrition information, but the typical restaurant burger without all the gunk is about 400 calories (leave off the bun, and you'll save about 125 calories).

Not on the Program

- Deluxe Bacon Double Cheeseburger
- Chicken Strips and Fries
- Chili Cheese Fries

APPLEBEE'S

www.applebees.com

This chain has a large enough menu to accommodate the nutrition-minded, and there are even some low-fat entrées that are clearly marked on the menu. Unfortunately, the menu also differs at different Applebee's, so you can't be 100 percent certain that your local branch will have all the lean offerings. Still, you can do well here if you read the menu carefully and ask them to hold the cheese where needed.

Top Picks
- Low-Fat Chicken Quesadilla—This is an appetizer but is a better choice as an entrée. The restaurant uses nonfat cheddar and mozzarella in the dish, which cuts down on the saturated fat.
- Most salads—Ordinarily I wouldn't recommend these; however, you can order half sizes, which makes them a healthier pick. Still, some of the salads will need some adjustments (such as getting the chef to leave off or limit the rice noodles in the Oriental Chicken Salad and the bleu cheese crumbles on the Steakhouse Salad). Ask for the dressing on the side.
- Sizzling Stir-Fry with Chicken
- Low-Fat Grilled Whitefish with Mango Salsa—A dish with less than 5 grams of fat.
- Honey Grilled Salmon—Watch out, though, for the side dishes, such as the garlic bread that it's served with.
- Honey Grilled Chicken—Ditto.
- Fajitas—This is a fine choice as long as you forgo the extras such as cheese, sour cream, and guacamole that Applebee's serves on the side.

Not on the Program
- Fried Chicken Salad
- Chicken Fried Chicken
- Anything with Alfredo (cream sauce) in the title
- Oversized steaks
- Sandwiches—They're all cheesy; however, if they will make you a simple smoked turkey or ham sandwich with mustard, go for it.

ARBY'S

www.arbys.com

This enduring chain has some of the healthiest options of any fast-food restaurant. But you also have to be careful: some of the items on the menu that sound as though they may be low (or at least lower) in calories really aren't. Conversely, some that sound foreboding are actually okay choices.

Top Picks
Sandwiches
- Light Grilled Chicken (280 calories)
- Light Roast Chicken Deluxe (260 calories)
- Light Roast Turkey Deluxe (260 calories)

Those are the best and most obvious choices, but also okay are:

- Junior Roast Beef sandwich—It's aimed at kids, but if you really want roast beef, Arby's specialty, this is a good one to go for (310 calories).
- Arby's Melt with Cheddar Roast Beef Sandwich—Surprised? So was I, but because the sandwich is relatively small, it's also relatively low in calories (340 calories). Hold the sauce and ask for the au jus, which has only 5 calories.
- Hot Ham 'N Swiss sandwich (340 calories)

Salads
- Roast Chicken (160 calories)
- Grilled Chicken (210 calories)
- Garden—Get the calorie-reduced Buttermilk Ranch Dressing (total: 130 calories).

Breakfast
Arby's is also open for breakfast, and while I don't really endorse it, if you must go, get the Sourdough with Ham sandwich. It's the selection with the smallest amount of calories (220) and least saturated fat (only 1.5 grams).

Not on the Program

- Big Montana Roast Beef Sandwich—The name alone should clue you in (630 calories).
- Chicken Bacon 'N Swiss (610 calories)
- Chicken Cordon Bleu (630 calories)
- Grilled Chicken Deluxe; Roast Chicken Club— These sandwiches both run between 450 and 630 calories.
- Sub Sandwiches and Market Fresh Sandwiches— Some have as many as 880 calories!

AU BON PAIN ★

aubonpain.com

You really don't have any excuse for eating poorly at Au Bon Pain. It has an incredibly varied menu and plenty of healthy options. Best of all, if you like, you can create your own sandwiches here so that there will be no nasty surprises (such as a 300-calorie special sauce) lurking between the bread.

Top Picks

Sandwiches:

- Your best bet here is the "make your own" sandwich. Go for lean meats, multigrain breads (as opposed to the croissants or focaccia), skip the oily condiments, and ask for it piled high with vegetables. You can also order half sandwiches here.
- If you are determined to have a premade sandwich, go for the Thai Chicken (490 calories) or Honey Smoked Turkey (540 calories).

Soups and Stews:

This is an excellent category to choose from— every selection is under 300 calories, and many of the stews and soups have very little fat (save for the Lobster Bisque and Chowders). The soups are generally high in sodium, so if you have high blood pressure or are on a salt-restricted diet for any reason, these—except for the reduced-sodium

Mediterranean Pepper Soup—might not be your best choices. The best of the best:

- Garden Vegetable (40 calories)
- French Onion (80 calories)
- Chicken Noodle (90 calories)
- Chicken Florentine (170 calories)
- French Moroccan Tomato Lentil (110 calories)
- Curried Rice and Lentil (100 calories)
- Black Bean (170 calories)
- Classic Chili with Beans (190 calories)
- Chicken Stew (230 calories)
- Chicken Chili (210 calories)
- Beef Stew (210 calories)

TIP: Soups and stews that have beans and legumes, such as lentils, are a great choice because they are high in fiber.

Salads:

The key here is to order the right dressing. Au Bon Pain offers several reduced-calorie options, all with less than 110 calories per two tablespoons: Fat-Free Raspberry, Lite Ranch, Lite Vinaigrette, Lite Honey Mustard, and Thai Peanut (not technically "reduced" but naturally low in calories). Next, pick salads that don't have a lot of fatty extras, such as the Garden, Mediterranean Chicken, or Charbroiled Salmon Filet Salad.

Breakfast

- Yogurt & Fruit Cups (310 calories)
- Oatmeal Bar—If you're on the run, this is not a bad choice (150 calories), and it has a fair amount (4 grams) of fiber.
- Cholesterol and Fat Free Eggs—Real eggs (if your cholesterol is not elevated) are fine too, but if you can't get them without all the extras (cheese, bacon, bagel), this 25-calorie selection is a good choice.
- Lowfat Triple Berry Muffin (290 calories)

Not on the Program
Sandwiches:

All the premade sandwiches and wraps are fairly caloric, but especially beware of the Chicken, Ham and Cambozola; Roast Beef and Pepperoncini; and Turkey, Ham, and Provolone sandwiches: they're over 1,000 calories each!

Salads:

If you choose the right dressing, all the salads are reasonable, but it's probably best not to order these fattier choices:

- Chicken Caesar Salad
- Tuna Salad
- Cobb Salad
- Mozzarella and Red Pepper Salad

Breakfast
- Raisin Bran Muffin—It sounds healthy and, fiber-wise, with 10 grams, it is. But it also has 520 calories and 6 grams of saturated fat—a lot for a little muffin that may not even keep you satisfied till lunch.
- Apple Spice Muffin (510 calories)—Ditto.
- Egg & Bagel with Cheese & Bacon (560 calories)

BAJA FRESH ★

This Mexican fast-food chain definitely gets an "E" for effort. Actually, "fast food" might be a little bit of a misnomer: because the chain uses all fresh ingredients and cooks everything to order. They make a point of warning customers that there may be a bit of a wait before they are served, but I've found it's not much of a wait at all. Baja Fresh doesn't use any lard in its food, a big plus as far as I'm concerned.

At the time of this writing, Baja Fresh was test-marketing several low-fat entrées. I'm not including them here since whether they were going to become regular features on the menu was still up in the air. But you should also know that Baja Fresh is very amenable to special orders. If you want grilled fish on your salad, or if you prefer your dishes without cheese, they're happy to oblige. The healthy choices are so abundant that you shouldn't have any trouble ignoring the unhealthy ones.

Top Picks

- Baja Style Tacos—The charbroiled chicken and shrimp tacos have only 190 calories each and a scant amount of saturated fat; even the char-broiled steak taco comes in at 220 calories and 2 grams saturated fat.
- Charbroiled Fish Taco—This taco is topped with avocado salsa, which pushes up its calorie count to 260. For a less calorific taco, ask them to leave off the sauce.

TIP: Soft tacos are often made with two tortillas. Ask that yours be made with one, and if that makes it hard to eat, use a knife and fork.

- Taco Chilito (320 calories)—Both the steak and chicken chilitos (open-faced tacos) are reason-able, but hold the sour cream.
- Baja Ensalada (310 calories chicken; 360 calo-ries fish—dressing not included). Have it with a little vinaigrette or ranch dressing but without the fried tortilla strips on top. To keep it really lean, dress it with fat-free salsa.
- Fajitas—Fine if you eat only the meat or chicken with grilled peppers and onions. Add in the rice, beans, sour cream, and guacamole, and the calo-ries reach into the stratosphere.
- Assemble your own platter—Baja Fresh offers everything you need to make a healthy meal à la carte. Choose among side orders of: pinto beans (320 calories); rice (280 calories); onions, pepper,

and chiles (110 calories); grilled green onions (called *cebollitas*—40 calories); charbroiled steak (210 calories); charbroiled chicken (230 calories); and shrimp (150 calories).

Not on the Program

- Burritos (upward of 830 calories)—Unless you special-order them without cheese and sour cream and keep to chicken and beans or beans and rice with pico de gallo. Definitely stay away from the Burrito Dos Manos—a burrito for two hands, which has to mean trouble! *Unless* you split it with someone, which is actually a good way to go.
- Taquitos (upward of 710 calories)
- Tostadas (1,140 calories)
- Enchiladas (upward of 780 calories)
- Quesadillas (upward of 1,180 calories)

BENIHANA ★

www.benihana.com

At this Japanese restaurant, known for its entertaining teppan table cooking, you can actually watch the chef to see how much oil he's putting in your food. Will he be amenable to using less? Definitely ask. If all else fails, stick to the dishes listed below.

Top Picks

- Benihana Delight—A combination of chicken and shrimp.
- Benihana Marina—Shrimp, calamari, and ocean scallops.
- Hibachi Chicken, Shrimp, or Scallops
- Teriyaki Chicken
- Sushi Combination
- Sashimi Dinner
- Japanese Onion Soup—This flavorful broth comes with the dinners, and while Benihana doesn't provide nutrition information, my guess is

that it is superlow in calories. You might even want to have two bowls and skip the salad that also comes with the dinner.

Not on the Program
- Any kind of tempura dish
- Fried tofu
- Hibachi Chateaubriand

BENNIGAN'S

www.bennigans.com

Traditionally, pub food has never been what you'd call health food, and it still packs a pretty good artery-clogging punch. But to its credit, the Irish-themed Bennigan's has made an effort to include some leaner selections on its menu. It may take some navigating between the deep-fried fish and jumbo burgers, but you'll find them.

Top Picks
- Chicken Noodle Soup—It's not on the menu everyday, but it is a good pick and a lot better than the other soups, which are more caloric.
- Bennigan's Club Salad—A good choice if you get them to hold the cheese and choose one of the lighter dressings (fat-free honey Dijon or lite Italian).
- Ahi Tuna Steak Salad
- Grilled Salmon Caesar Salad—Perfect if it can be ordered without the Parmesan cheese and croutons and with dressing on the side.
- Boca Burger—Usually served with cheese, but I'm sure they'll leave it off if asked.
- O'Malley's Pork Chops . . . especially if you split it. The entrée comes with two chops, more than you probably need.
- Chicken Stir-Fry—One of Bennigan's leaner dishes.
- Chicken Platter—Served with rice and broccoli.

Not on the Program
- Pub Starters—There's really not one of them that's isn't high in fat.
- Kilkenny's Country Chicken Salad—Sounds harmless enough, but the chicken is breaded and fried.
- Burgers
- Ribs
- Steak dishes
- Fish dishes—Most are fried or pan-sautéed.
- Sandwiches—They tend to be overstuffed and fatty.

BIG APPLE BAGEL
www.babholdings.com

Bagels, as you're probably well aware, generally pack a lot of calories (unless they're small, and hardly anyone makes them small anymore). Big Apple's tend to be about 380 calories each. So keep that in mind when ordering.

Top Picks
Soups:

They're all terrific choices. Even the most caloric one (Cheese and Bacon) tops out at only 310 calories.

- French Onion (60 calories)
- Split Pea with Ham (90 calories)
- Beef Barley Mushroom (100 calories)
- Garden Vegetable (110 calories)

Sandwiches:
- Bagel with Lite Cream Cheese—Ask for just a touch of cream cheese, not a glob, and consider having a half bagel instead of a whole one.

TIP: Try a kaiser roll instead of a bagel—they have about half the calories.

- Grilled Chicken—Hold the mayo.
- Classic Turkey—Likewise.

Not on the Program

- Roma Italian Sub
- All-American Duo Sub
- Breakfast BLT
- Jumbo Muffins

BIG BOY

www.bigboy.com

Is it my imagination, or has Big Boy, this restaurant's eponymous icon, lost a few pounds? In any case, the establishment known for hamburgers with names such as "Brawny Lad" has made a concerted effort to add healthy selections to its menu. There's even a nutrition chart on the back of the menu so you can get specifics before you make your selection.

Top Picks

- Soup, Salad, and Fruit Bar—While this is an all-you-can-eat buffet, you can still eat healthfully if you practice portion control—and, of course, make the right choices. Go for light soups such as Cabbage Soup (skip the soup if the only offerings are creamy), fresh vegetables, and the lo-cal Ranch or fat-free Italian dressing. Forgo the prepared salads, cheese, meat, and other fatty extras such as croutons.
- Chicken Breast Salad—If you're going to eat the accompanying roll, leave off the *faux*-butter spread that comes with it.
- Turkey Pita
- Chargrilled Chicken Breast—Hold the mayo.
- Chicken 'n Vegetable Stir Fry
- Vegetable Stir Fry
- Broiled Cod
- Cajun Cod
- Spaghetti Marinara

TIP: These last five entrées come with a roll *and* (in most cases) a baked potato. That's a lot of extra starch you probably don't need. Choose one or the other (and neither if you're having pasta).

- Frozen Yogurt—A nice fat-free finisher to your meal, but be aware that it contains a lot of sugar.

Breakfast
- Two eggs—Substitute the tomatoes for the potatoes and limit yourself to one piece of toast.
- Scrambled Egg Beaters
- Plain Egg Beaters Omelette
- Vegetarian Egg Beaters Omelette

Not on the Program
- Burgers
- Super Salads
- Sandwiches (except those mentioned above)
- Fried fish entrées
- Chicken Wisconsin—Smothered with Wisconsin's pride (cheese, that is).

Breakfast
- Cinnamon French Toast
- Regular Omelettes
- Belgian Waffles
- All-You-Can-Eat Breakfast and Fruit Bar

BLIMPIE

www.blimpie.com

Submarine sandwiches, the specialty here, are by nature oversized and tend to be high in calories. But one of the great things about these particular subs is that they're made to order so you can get them the way you like. For instance, as a rule, the grilled subs, if you order them off the menu, tend to be higher in calories than even the regular subs. If you simply ask the counterperson to leave off the cheese, you'll get a healthier sandwich. If you prefer to just order off the menu as is, here's what to (and not to) go for.

Top Picks

Sandwiches:

- VegiMax Hot Sub (395 calories)
- MexiMax Hot Sub (425 calories)
- Seafood Cold Sub (355 calories)
- Turkey Cold Sub (425 calories)
- Ham and Cheese Cold Sub (436 calories)

Soups:

All the selections are a great choice, but if you're looking for a low-low-calorie bowl, the Garden Vegetable Soup (80) and Vegetable Beef (80) are your best picks.

Salads:

- Antipasto Salad (244 calories)
- Chef Salad (212 calories)
- Seafood Salad (122 calories)
- Tuna Salad (261 calories)

TIP: Remember, it's the dressing that really counts. Unless your local Blimpie offers a low-cal variety, use dressing sparingly.

Not on the Program

- Wraps—These range from 650 to more than 800 calories.
- Grilled Subs—Ditto, unless you get them made to your own conscientious specifications.
- Cole Slaw, Macaroni Salad, Mustard Potato Salad—Forget the sides, which tend to be fatty.

BOB EVANS

www.bobevans.com

Some restaurants have everything you need to dine healthfully on their menus—they just don't necessarily put those items together in a healthful way. Bob Evans is one of those places, although it does have a few entrées that you can order "as is" and do okay. Really read the menu thoroughly, and all the smart options should jump out at you.

Top Picks
Breakfast
- Lite Sausage Breakfast—Beside the reduced-fat sausage, this consists of Egg Beaters, fresh fruit, and dry wheat toast.
- Fruit Plate—Pass on the biscuits that accompany it and order toast instead.
- Strawberry Yogurt
- Oatmeal
- Two eggs—If you don't have elevated cholesterol, this is always a good breakfast choice, but you'll need to opt out of the potatoes and biscuits. Order a dry English muffin instead.

Lunch
- Fresh Fruit and Yogurt Plate
- Classic Bean Soup
- Beef Vegetable Soup
- Bob Evans Combo—Choose soup and the Garden Salad or the salad and a plain baked potato.
- Grilled Chicken Stir-fry
- Grilled Chicken Club Sandwich—They'll make it without the bacon and cheese; skip the fries.

Dinner
- Turkey—This may take some creative ordering. It comes with dressing, side dishes, and gravy. Try to get them to serve the turkey breast without all the extras, order a side salad or one of the vegetable choices, and you're in business.
- Grilled Chicken Stir-fry
- Vegetable Stir-fry
- Grilled Garden Vegetables and a Baked Potato (plain)
- Grilled New Orleans–Style Catfish—It's typically served with two pieces of fish, but you can also get it with just one.

Not on the Program
Breakfast
- Farmer's Breakfast—Eggs, meat, fries, and pancakes—in other words, way too much food!
- Pot Roast Hash
- Sausage Gravy Breakfast
- Bob Evans Skillets

Lunch
- Wildfire Pulled Pork Sandwich
- Chicken Broccoli Alfredo
- Raspberry Grilled Chicken Salad—Deceptively innocuous-sounding, it actually contains bleu cheese and bacon.
- Wildfire Chicken Salad—Fried chicken with tortilla strips and cheese. Need I say more?

Dinner
- Burgers
- Sirloin Steak Tips and Noodles
- Country Fried Steak
- Steak Monterey—It's topped with cheese, making this a real cholesterol fest.

BOJANGLES'

www.bojangles.com

Fried chicken and biscuits are the specialty here, so the pickings are kind of slim if you're hoping for a moderate-fat meal. Still, you should be able to find a few things to tide you over.

Top Picks
Sandwiches:
- Cajun Filet—Leaving off the mayonnaise reduces the calorie count of this sandwich from 437 to 337 and knocks off 11 grams of fat.
- Grilled Filet—Again, eschew the mayo, and the sandwich will be a lot more healthful.

Side Dishes:

Pick and choose among these to make a meal:

- Corn on the Cob (140 calories)
- Cajun Pintos (110 calories)
- Marinated Cole Slaw (136 calories)
- Green Beans (25 calories)

Not on the Program
- Fried Chicken
- Biscuit Sandwiches

BOSTON MARKET ★

www.bostonmarket.com

There is an abundance of healthful choices at Boston Market, including vegetable side dishes that aren't swimming in fat—a rarity in the take-out world. There are many things on the menu that can tip your daily calorie balance, but there are so many lean dishes to counter them that there's really no excuse for not eating conscientiously here.

Top Picks
Sandwiches:
- Marinated Grilled Chicken, no mayo (470 calories)
- Chicken, no cheese or sauce (400 calories)
- Turkey, no cheese or sauce (400 calories)

Entrées:
- 1/4 White Meat Chicken (170 calories)
- Skinless Rotisserie Turkey Breast (170 calories)
- Marinated Grilled Chicken (230 calories per breast)

Side Dishes:
- Butternut Squash (150 calories)
- Green Beans (70 calories)
- New Potatoes (130 calories)
- Rice Pilaf (140 calories)

- Steamed Vegetables (30 calories)
- Fruit Salad (70 calories)

Soups:
- Chicken Tortilla Soup, no toppings (80 calories)
- Turkey Tortilla Soup, no toppings (70 calories)
- Chicken Noodle Soup (100 calories)

Not on the Program
Salads and Sandwiches:
- Oriental Grill Chicken Salad with Dressing and Noodles (660 calories)
- Southwest Grill Chicken Salad with Dressing and Chips (890 calories)
- Open-Faced Meatloaf Sandwich with Potatoes and Gravy (730 calories)
- Turkey Bacon Club Sandwich (770 calories)
- BBQ Grilled Chicken Sandwich (830 calories)

Entrées:
- Chicken Pot Pie (750 calories)
- ½ Chicken with skin (590 calories)

Side Dishes:
- Cole Slaw (300 calories)
- Old-Fashioned Potato Salad (200 calories)
- Tortellini Salad (350 calories)
- Sweet potato casserole (280 calories)

BRUEGGER'S BAGELS

www.brueggers.com

While big bagels can be high in calories, they are still better for you than pastries with saturated fat and/or lots of sugar, such as croissants and cinnamon buns. But also be aware that when you have a bagel sandwich for lunch, like the specialties offered by Bruegger's, you'll have already rung up more than 300 calories worth of bread even before you decide on what you want for your filling. Consider paring down your sandwich by removing the top half of the bagel and eating it open-faced.

Top Picks

- Bagel with light cream cheese—Ask for a schmear, not an overload of cream cheese.
- Leonardo da Veggie Sandwich—Hold the Muenster cheese.
- Turkey Sandwich—Swap mustard for the mayo.
- Chicken Breast Sandwich
- Ham Deli Sandwich

Not on the Program

- Herby Turkey Sandwich
- Chicken Fajita Sandwich

BURGER KING

www.burgerking.com

Fortunately, the home of the Whopper is learning to accommodate customers who don't want a whopping serving of saturated fat for lunch. Did you know that if you went all out and ordered a Double Whopper with Cheese, a large order of fries, and a medium chocolate shake, you'd end up ingesting 2,360 calories and 61 grams of saturated fat? Looking at the numbers (to see more, check out the Burger King Web site) can really be a wake-up call. But there are now other options, so don't give into temptation; as the old Burger King ad says, have it your way—the healthy way.

Top Picks

- Chicken Caesar Salad—Skip the Caesar dressing and go for either the Fat-Free Ranch or Light Italian.
- Side Salad—Again, choose the calorie-conscious dressings.
- BK Veggie Burger with Reduced Fat Mayo (290 calories)

- Chicken Whopper Sandwich without mayo (420 calories)
- Baked Potato with chives (260 calories)

Breakfast

Not my favorite choice, but if you're in a jam:

- Sourdough Breakfast Sandwich with Ham, Egg, and Cheese—If possible, get them to leave off the cheese.

CALIFORNIA PIZZA KITCHEN

www.cpk.com

One of the advantages of this restaurant over the traditional pizzeria is that you get your own personal pizza, so you're not beholden to the desires of your dining companions. Moreover, it has so many toppings that you can really stack your pizza high with vegetables. In fact, you can order a pizza without cheese and still feel satisfied because there are so many other good toppings to be had. CPK also has many other dishes on the menu, so don't feel that pizza is your only option.

Top Picks

- Sedona White Corn Tortilla Soup
- Dakota Smashed Pea and Barley Soup
- Field Greens—All of the salads here come in both appetizer and meal sizes.
- Original Chopped Salad—This comes with salami, which you may or may not want to leave out depending on what you've eaten during the rest of the day.
- Tricolore Salad—This is essentially a pizza with a salad on top instead of tomato sauce and mozzarella.
- Traditional Cheese Pizza
- Vegetarian with Japanese Eggplant Pizza

- Margherita Pizza
- Grilled Garlic Shrimp Pizza

TIP: Consider having half a pizza (either splitting it with your dining companion or taking half home) and rounding out your meal with a half salad or soup.

- Broccoli/Sun-dried Tomato Fusilli—Hold the cheese.
- Marsala Marinara Linguini—Ditto.
- Tomato Basil Spaghettini—Add grilled chicken breast if you like.
- Grilled Rosemary Chicken Sandwich—This is a nice option; however, it's served on focaccia bread, which can be pretty calorie-dense. Consider taking the top off the sandwich.

Not on the Program
- Smoked Bacon and Gorgonzola Chopped Salad
- B.L.T. Pizza
- Pear and Gorgonzola Pizza
- Sweet & Spicy Italian Sausages Pizza
- Sicilian Pizza
- Chicken-Tequila Fettuccine
- Fettucine with Garlic Cream Sauce

CAPTAIN D'S SEAFOOD

www.captainds.com

It's nice to find a place that believes fish doesn't have to be fried to taste good. Some of the Captain D's branches (although unfortunately not all) offer broiled entrées. While oil is usually used in the broiling process, the seafood will still be a lot less fatty than if it spent time in the deep-fat fryer.

Top Picks
- Anything on the Captain's Broiler menu (where available)

- Broiled Pacific Northwest Salmon
- Broiled New Zealand Orange Roughy
- Broiled Chicken Sandwich—Forgo the fries.
- Broiled Whitefish Sandwich—Ditto.
- Baked Potato

Not on the Program
- Any of the fried fish or chicken meals

CARL'S JR.

www.carlsjr.com

Carl's Jr. advertises itself as the place to get messy, gargantuan burgers, so, as you might imagine, the chain's main focus is on the splurge. It has, however, given a nod to the health-conscious by adding a couple of more modest items to the menu. You won't have a lot of choices here, but at least you'll have a few.

Top Picks
- Charbroiled BBQ Chicken Sandwich (290 calories)
- Charbroiled Chicken Salad-to-go (200 calories)—The calorie count will go up only slightly if you choose the Fat Free Italian Dressing or Fat Free French Dressing.
- Garden Salad-to-go (50 calories)—Ditto on the dressing.
- Plain Potato without margarine (290 calories)

Breakfast
- Scrambled Eggs (180 calories)

Not on the Program
- Any of the hamburgers, which range in calories from 590 to 920 (the Double Western Bacon Cheeseburger is a veritable heart attack waiting to happen)
- Crispy Chicken Sandwiches
- Chicken Stars—The calories are low (260 for 5 pieces, but the fat is high: 16 grams).

Breakfast
- Breakfast Burrito (550 calories)
- Croissant Sunrise Sandwich (359 calories)

CARROWS

www.carrows.com

This is the type of restaurant that may not offer many predesigned low-calorie and low-fat dishes but has everything needed to create a healthy meal. You'll just need to be creative in designing and be assertive in asking for the food you want.

Top Picks
Breakfast
- Two eggs and toast—Ask for fruit rather than hash browns. For your toast, Carrows serves Promise, a non–trans fat margarine.
- Oatmeal
- Cold cereal with fruit

Lunch
- Garden burger—Skip the fries and cole slaw and ask for a dinner salad instead.
- Plain grilled chicken breast or plain roast turkey sandwich—Neither of these is on the menu in this pared-down state, but you can probably get them to leave off the fixin's.
- Noncreamy soups

Dinner
- Broiled Salmon
- Plain grilled chicken breast—Again, not on the menu, but surely they can omit the sauce that usually comes with it.
- Old-Fashioned Spaghetti—Get the marinara sauce; hold the Parmesan.

Not on the Program
Breakfast
- Omelettes

- Skillet Eggs
- Pancakes and waffles

Lunch
- Any of the Mile-High Sandwiches
- Chicken Quesadilla and Baja Caesar Salad

Dinner
- Chicken Pot Pie
- Chicken Fettuccine Primavera
- Smoky Mountain BBQ Ribs

CHART HOUSE

www.chart-house.com

This is a great place to go when you know your dining companions are hankering for a steak or something that you are not going to eat. They can have their filet mignon while you dine happily on one of the many seafood selections.

Top Picks
Appetizers:
- Shrimp Cocktail
- Seared Peppered Ahi Tuna
- Chart House Salad or, if available, the salad bar—If you choose the latter (which you can also get as an entrée), watch out for the greasy croutons and big hunks of bread.

Entrées:
- Any of the fish dishes, cooked to your specifications—Use your best judgment: some of the fish dishes come with fattening sauces, so it's probably best to ask for plain, grilled fish with a slice of lemon.
- Pan-Seared Sea Scallops
- Alaskan King Crab Legs—Nix the accompanying butter.
- Dungeness Crab Clusters—Order them steamed instead of garlic style.

Sides:

- Baked Potato—Just be wise about what you dress it up with. Hot sauce or a low-cal dressing, if they have it, is a good choice.
- Steamed Asparagus

Not on the Program

- Appetizers, except for those listed above
- Lobster Bisque
- Clam Chowder—This creamy New England–style soup is award-winning but not waist-thinning.
- Coconut Crunchy Shrimp
- Prime Rib
- Australian Lobster Tail—It's baked with butter.

CHI-CHI'S

www.chi-chis.com

This is one of the few chain Mexican restaurants that offers grilled items, so kudos to them. Still, be careful. As per usual in Mexican-style eateries, there are lots of fatty extras such as cheese, refried beans, sour cream, and guacamole.

Top Picks

- Low Fat Chicken Soft Taco—With 24 percent of its calories from fat, this dish meets the definition of low fat, yet it still has 18 grams (and 680 calories). That's not too bad for Mexican food, but be aware that you're not getting a super-low-fat meal.
- Low Fat Chicken Enchiladas—The same goes for these, which weigh in with 695 calories and 22 grams of fat.
- Grilled Blackened or Mesquite Chicken
- Grilled Garlic Shrimp
- Santa Fe Chicken
- Fajitas
- Grilled or Blackened Chicken Sandwich
- Santa Fe–Style Grilled Chicken Salad—Only if they'll hold the cheese.

Not on the Program

- Texas Nachos
- Outrageous Burrito
- Tortilla-Crusted Chicken Fajitas
- Seafood Enchilada—It's "swimming" (the restaurant's word) in sherry cream sauce and cheese.

CHICK-FIL-A

www.chickfila.com

One of the biggest chicken restaurant chains in the country, Chick-fil-A doesn't automatically drown their chicken in fat, as do some of their competitors. It has some guilt-free options—just remember that adding greasy sauces will raise the calorie count substantially.

Top Picks

Sandwiches:

- Chick-fil-A Chargrilled Chicken Sandwich, no butter (240 calories)
- Chargrilled Chicken, no bun (100 calories)
- Chargrilled Chicken Cool Wrap (390 calories)— The wraps are almost as high in calories as the fried chicken sandwich; however, they have half the fat.
- Spicy Chicken Cool Wrap (390 calories)

TIP: If you want to add a sauce, choose either the barbecue or honey mustard sauces, both of which are fat free.

Sides:

- Hearty Breast of Chicken Soup (100 calories)
- Salad (80 calories)—Light Italian and Fat Free Dijon Honey Mustard Dressings are offered.
- Small Carrot and Raisin Salad (130 calories)

Not on the Program

- Chick-fil-A Chick-N-Strips Salad
- Chick-fil-A Chicken Salad Sandwich

- Chick-fil-A Chicken Sandwich
- Chicken Deluxe Sandwich
- Cole Slaw

CHILI'S GRILL & BAR FAMILY RESTAURANT

www.chilis.com

Chili's has its fair share of fat traps—it's the kind of place where people go to indulge with abandon. The restaurant, though, makes it a little easier to side step calorie land mines by offering some dishes that it calls "guiltless" entrées.

Top Picks

- Guiltless Grill Pita—It's stuffed with grilled chicken and topped with low-fat Ranch dressing.
- Guiltless Chicken Sandwich
- Guiltless Chicken Platter
- Margarita Grilled Tuna—Ask if you can get it plain, without the aïoli and other toppings.
- Lettuce Wraps—Filled with grilled chicken and a good choice if you avoid the peanut dipping sauce.
- Soup and dinner salad—Chili's has a good choice of low-fat dressings.

TIP: There are chicken fajitas on the menu here, which are a good choice if (and only if) you can get them served very plain and without a lot of oil. Ask how the fajitas are prepared; then make your decision based on how lean they're willing to make them for you.

Not on the Program

- All appetizers except Lettuce Wraps
- Sandwiches
- Baby Back Ribs
- Steaks
- Salads except those mentioned above
- Quesadillas
- Grilled Shrimp Alfredo
- Big Mouth Burgers

CHUCK E. CHEESE'S

www.chuckecheese.com

Since kids love Chuck E. Cheese's, sometimes parents just have to go along for the ride. The menu is small, and so, unfortunately, are your choices.

Top Picks
- Salad bar with Lite Ranch or Kraft Catalina dressing
- Two slices of cheese pizza—This is actually a better choice than the healthy-sounding Grilled Chicken Sub. The latter is 740 calories, the pizza 330.

Not on the Program
- Ham and Cheese Sandwich
- Italian Sub
- Hot Dog

CHURCH'S CHICKEN

www.churchs.com

Traditional southern-fried chicken with all the fixin's is the mainstay here, which doesn't leave you a lot of options. Think plain vegetables, and if you don't mind the mess (I think it's well worth it), trim your chicken of skin and fat.

Top Picks
- Chicken with the skin and batter removed—Church's gives you the impetus to take off the fried skin by providing nutrition data about "naked chicken." According to its calculations, a breast with the skin removed has 145 calories and 5.5 grams of fat, a significant reduction from the 230 calories and 16 grams of fat the breast has with the skin still on.
- Mashed Potatoes and Gravy (90 calories)
- Collard Greens (25 calories)

- Corn on the Cob (139 calories)
- Cajun Rice (130 calories)

Not on the Program

It's not the calories so much as the fat that makes these bad choices. Here's what I mean:

- Fried Chicken (a thigh has 16 grams of fat)
- Chicken Fried Steak with White Gravy (28 grams of fat)
- Honey Butter Biscuits (16 grams of fat)
- Okra (16 grams of fat)
- Sweet Corn Nuggets (12 grams of fat)
- Creamy Jalapeño Sauce and Honey Mustard Sauce—Both have 11 grams of fat, while the BBQ Sauce and Sweet and Sour Sauce have 0.

THE COOKERY

This diner-style eatery doesn't have a special menu or even special entrées for those concerned about fat and calories. That means you're stuck with the regular menu, though fortunately it has a few reasonable offerings. You may need to ask for some special considerations here to make your meal leaner, but since the food is cooked to order, that shouldn't be a problem.

Top Picks

- Sensational Soup and Salad Bar—Of course, it depends what the soup of the day is, but if it's not a cream soup, this is a good choice. The salad bar also offers you some control over what goes onto your plate. The entrée salads tend to have high-calorie extras such as cheese and croutons mixed in. Fat-free dressing is available.
- Grilled Chicken Sandwich

With the following entrées, skip the garlic bread and order a plain baked potato rather than fries:

- Chicken Teriyaki
- Chicken Stir Fry
- Vegetable Stir Fry
- Grilled Tilapia Filet

Not on the Program
- Country Classics Entrées—These tend to be fried, cheesy, or made from fat-marbled meats.
- Burgers
- Sandwiches (except the Grilled Chicken Sandwich mentioned above)

COUSINS SUBS ★

www.cousinssubs.com

Submarine sandwiches can be exorbitantly high in fat and calories, so it's important to order with care at a sub shop. Cousins tries to make it easier by providing a lineup of sandwiches and soups with 6 grams of fat or less.

Top Picks
- Cold Subs: Roast Beef, Ham, Club Sub, Turkey Breast, Cold Veggie
- Hot Subs: Chicken Breast
- Mini Subs: Ham, Turkey Breast

TIP: These subs are low-fat, but only because they're made without mayo and cheese. Make sure when you order them that's it's clear you want them without the fatty extras.

- Soups: Chicken Noodle, Tomato Basil, Red Beans and Rice

Not on the Program
- Italian Special Sub
- Philly Cheese Steak Hot Sub
- Tuna Mini Sub
- Soups: Chicken with Wild Rice, Cheese Broccoli, Vegetable Beef

CULVER'S

www.culvers.com

As you'd imagine, if you're eating at the home of ButterBurgers and renowned frozen custard, it's a good idea to use caution. But fortunately Culver's menu isn't all burgers and sweets; it also contains several acceptable items that you can feel comfortable ordering. At first glance I might have dismissed it as another cholesterol-loving burger joint, but that just goes to show that you really have to pay attention to the menu.

Top Picks

Sandwiches:
- Grilled Chicken (370 calories)—They serve mayo on the side; ask for mustard instead.
- Beef Pot Roast Sandwich (330 calories)— Unexpectedly moderate in calories.
- Corn Dog (260 calories)—It has more than 100 fewer calories than the hot dog. Go figure.

Salads:
- Chicken Caesar Salad (280 calories)
- Chicken Parmesan Salad (295 calories)
- Hot 'n Spicy Chicken Salad (290 calories)
- Side Salad

TIP: Culver's offers a few low-calorie dressings (fat-free Italian, fat-free toasted sesame, and reduced-calorie ranch) but also serves most of its salads with cheese. Ask if they'll leave it off.

Soups:
Soups are one of your best choices here. They're all fairly healthy and low in calories and saturated fat except for the four listed below.

Not on the Program
- Any of the ButterBurgers (461–780 calories)
- Chili Cheese Dog (500 calories, 320 of them from fat)

- Fried Chicken and Fish dinners (the fish and chips has 910 calories)
- Philly Steak Sandwich (500 calories)
- Tuna Sourdough Sandwich (600 calories)
- Soups high in saturated fat: Broccoli Cheese; Chicken Pot Pie; Potato Au Gratin; Wisconsin Cheese

DAIRY QUEEN

www.dairyqueen.com

On this limited menu of classic burger joint fare, there are a few sensible items that won't require you to pay penance the rest of the day. I think it's worth noting that if you are going out for ice cream, Dairy Queen is one of the better choices. Their specialty soft serve ice cream contains considerably less fat and calories than a premium ice cream such as Häagen-Dazs. A small cup of vanilla, for instance, has only 3 grams of saturated fat. Try, though, to avoid all the extras such as candy mix-ins, fudge sauce, and cookies.

Top Picks
- Grilled Chicken Sandwich (240 calories)
- Grilled Chicken Salad with fat-free Italian (230 calories)
- BBQ Pork Sandwich (280 calories)—Lower in saturated fat than the hamburger.
- BBQ Beef Sandwich (300 calories)—Likewise.

Not on the Program
- DQ Ultimate Burger
- Chicken Breast Fillet Sandwich
- Crispy Chicken Salad

D'ANGELO SANDWICH SHOPS ★

www.dangelo.com

Now, here's a fast-food restaurant that has gone out of its way to service customers interested in preserving their health. The company even has a guide to eating healthfully at D'Angelo on its Web site.

Top Picks

- D'Lite Sandwiches—There are seven of these reduced-calorie sandwiches on the menu, ranging from Chicken Stir Fry to Turkey Cranberry. None of the sandwiches has more than 7 grams of fat, and they are also low in sodium (using unsalted turkey is one way the restaurant keeps the salt content down).
- Grilled Chicken Pokket Sandwich—Also low in fat.
- Classic Veggie Pokket Sandwich, No Cheese—Ditto.
- Soups—Especially the Vegetable, Chicken Noodle, French Onion, and Minestrone.
- All Salads with Fat-Free Caesar dressing—Except, ironically, the Caesar Salad, which is high in fat and calories even with the fat-free dressing.

Not on the Program

- Regular Subs
- Wraps

DEL TACO

www.deltaco.com

While the emphasis here is on Mexican food, Del Taco also serves classic fast food such as burgers and fries. There's nothing really aimed at the health-conscious diner so just try to go for the least objectionable items.

Top Picks

- Soft Taco (160 calories)
- Bean and Cheese Burrito, Red or Green (270–280 calories)
- Rice Cup (140 calories)
- Beans 'n Cheese Cup (260 calories)

Breakfast
- Breakfast Burrito (250 calories)

Not on the Program
- Any of the Macho Burritos (930–1170 calories)
- Quesadillas (upward of 490 calories)
- Deluxe Chicken Salad (740 calories)

Breakfast
- Macho Bacon and Egg Burrito (1,030 calories)

DENNY'S ★

www.dennys.com

Denny's has about 1,700 restaurants, and it's a good place to stop when you're on the road; there are always always several things on the menu that you can eat. Denny's has developed selections under the name "Fit Fare," which contain less than 15 grams of fat. That, at least, is the criterion it uses; however, many of the entrées are actually quite a bit lower in fat (and, most important, saturated fat).

Top Picks
- Grilled Chicken Breast Dinner (130 calories not including side dishes)
- Pot Roast Dinner with gravy (292 calories not including side dishes)
- Roast Turkey and Stuffing (388 calories not including side dishes)
- Turkey Breast Sandwich on multigrain bread (476 calories)
- Garden Salad Deluxe with Chicken Breast (264 calories)—Choose the Fat Free Ranch Dressing or Low Calorie Italian.
- Garden Salad Deluxe with Turkey and Ham (322 calories)—Ditto.

Side Dishes:
- Garden Salad (113 calories)

- Sliced Tomatoes (13 calories)
- Carrots in Honey Glaze (80 calories)
- Baked Potato, plain (220 calories)
- Vegetable Rice Pilaf (88 calories)
- Corn in Butter Sauce (120 calories)—They must add just a touch of butter, because this dish has only 4 grams of fat. The same goes for Green Peas in Butter Sauce (100 calories).
- Green Beans with Bacon (60 calories)
- Musselman's Applesauce (60 calories)

Breakfast
- SlimSlam without topping (438 calories)—One of Denny's most famous offerings is the 795-calorie Original Grand Slam, a coronary on a plate consisting of two hotcakes, two eggs, two strips of bacon, and two sausage links. It pares it down nicely in this variation, which includes two Egg Beaters, a slice of ham, and two hotcakes.
- Oatmeal (100 calories)
- Grits (80 calories)
- Bagel (235 calories)
- Fruit

Not on the Program
- Appetizers
- T-Bone Steak Dinner (860 calories)
- Fried Shrimp & Shrimp Scampi (346 calories and 20 g fat)
- Club Sandwich (718 calories)
- BBQ Chicken Sandwich (1072 calories)
- Bacon Cheddar Burger (875 calories)

Breakfast
- Big Texas Chicken Fajita Skillet (1,217 calories)
- Any of the "Slams" except the SlimSlam
- Breakfast Dagwood (1,251 calories)
- Fabulous French Toast (939 calories)

DOMINO'S PIZZA

www.dominos.com

As with pizza from any pizzeria, the key to ordering here is choosing the least offensive "style." Toppings, of course, count at Dominos, but you'll find that the type of crust you order makes a significant difference. Fatter crusts make for, well, you know.

Top Picks

- Thin Crust Pizza with vegetable toppings—One quarter of a medium-thick-crust pizza (with cheese only) has about 273 calories. Now compare that with an equivalent serving of the Deep Dish Cheese (482 calories) and the Classic Hand Tossed Cheese (374 calories)
- Barbeque Wings or Hot Wings—I'm not crazy about these, but Domino's menu is very limited, and these chicken wings are about 50 calories each. Just don't order sauce on the side, which will increase their fat count considerably.

Not on the Program

- Classic Hand-Tossed ExtravaganZZa Feast Pizza
- Classic Hand-Tossed Bacon Cheeseburger Feast Pizza
- Buffalo Chicken Kickers—They're fried.
- Cheesy Bread

DONATOS PIZZA

www.donatos.com

Even though the specialties here, pizza and subs, are two of the most fat-laden types of fast food you can get, it's still possible to have a meal here and not feel as though your next stop might be the cardiac ward. Donatos is a place, too, where your negotiating skills ("Can I have that without cheese, please?") will come in handy.

Top Picks
- Grilled Chicken Salad with Lite Italian Dressing (334 calories)
- Italian Chef Salad with Lite Italian Dressing (358 calories)

TIP: If you're contemplating getting the regular Italian dressing, keep in mind that 1½ ounces is 230 calories compared to 20 calories for the lite version.

- Ham and Cheese Sub with Lite Italian Dressing (534 calories)—All the better if you can be satisfied with half—the sandwich is fairly large.
- Individual Chicken Vegy Medley Original Pizza (500 calories)—Be sure that you get original crust, not traditional crust, which is thicker and higher in fat and calories.

Not on the Program
- Serious Meat, Serious Cheese, or the Works Pizzas
- Grilled Chicken Sub—When I saw that this sub had 786 calories and 43 grams of fat, I had to wonder what could possibly make a chicken sandwich so fattening. Bacon and two cheeses, as it turns out. If you can get the cook to make you a sub with just grilled chicken, vegetables, and lite dressing, by all means go for it.
- Steak and Cheese Sub (929 calories)

DUNKIN' DONUTS

www.dunkindonuts.com

You might wonder why I'd even include Dunkin' Donuts in this guide, because doughnuts, obviously, are not on the program. But this quick-stop (primarily) breakfast shop is so ubiquitous that I think its menu deserves a look. First, I want to point out something surprising: doughnuts do not have that many calories, especially compared to muffins or those monster cinnamon rolls that are now sold in every airport terminal. A Dunkin' Donuts glazed doughnut has 180 calories (cake doughnuts tend to have about 100 calories more, as do chocolate glazed doughnuts); its Coffee Cake Muffin has 710, and its Cinnamon Bun has 510.

I'm not telling you this to encourage you to eat doughnuts. A glazed doughnut may only have 180 calories, but it also has 15 grams of fat—and because Dunkin' Donuts uses partially hydrogenated soybean oil for cooking, that's unhealthy fat, to boot. On top of that is the fact that doughnuts don't contribute a lot of nutrients to your diet! But what I do want you to realize is that if you are going to indulge yourself on occasion, pick your poison well: there really is a difference among treats. Ideally, you'll have neither a doughnut, a big fatty muffin, nor a gargantuan cinnamon bun, because as you can see below, there are other options.

Top Picks
- Bagel—At about 340 calories, these are more energy dense than the doughnuts, but they have only a scant amount of saturated fat. Choose the lite cream cheese or ask for jam.
- English Muffin with Ham, Egg, and Cheese—You can't avoid having a little saturated fat with this pick (6 grams); however, you'll also be getting a good dose of vitamins and minerals from the egg, ham, and cheese. A doughnut may have fewer calories (this has 320), but it doesn't have nearly the nutritional value.

Not on the Program
- Reduced Fat Blueberry Muffin—The reduction in fat is all relative: The regular Blueberry Muffin has 17 grams of fat, this one has 13 grams, which is still too many.
- Muffins, especially the Chocolate Chip Muffin or Coffee Cake Muffin

EINSTEIN BROS' BAGELS

www.einsteinbros.com

Not surprisingly, many bagel shops limit your bread selection to bagels. Einstein Bros, though, has a little wider selection (which can help you cut back on calories) and offers some reduced-fat sandwiches.

Top Picks

- Build Your Own Bros Deli sandwich—Use the opportunity to order a smoked turkey breast, ham, or low-fat albacore tuna salad sandwich on twelve-grain bread. Forgo the accompanying chips and any fatty condiments such as mayo.
- Soups—Especially Homemade Chicken Noodle and Low Fat Minestrone.

Breakfast

- Scrambled eggs—These are usually cooked with cheese; ask for just plain scrambled eggs.
- Bagel with a reduced-fat schmear

Not on the Program

- The Cobbie Sandwich—Egg bread with turkey, bacon, avocado, and Gorgonzola cheese. In other words, a fat fest.
- Club Mex—Lots of cheese and bacon.

Breakfast

- Santa Fe Eggs—Sausage and cheese make this not a great way to start the day.

EL POLLO LOCO ★

www.elpolloloco.com

This is a great place to go if your dining companions want traditional Mexican with all the trappings but you want something lean. Although there are tacos and burritos on the menu, El Pollo Loco specializes in flame-broiled chicken, so it's the perfect compromise. If you're a vegetarian, you can also cobble together a good meal from El Pollo Loco's various side dishes.

Top Picks
- Flame-Broiled Chicken Breast (160 calories)
- Taco al Carbon (180 calories)
- Flame Broiled Chicken Salad Bowl (357 calories)—Light dressing is available.
- Small corn tortilla (32 calories)
- Pinto beans (185 calories)
- Spanish rice (130 calories)
- Corn cobbette (80 calories)
- Salsa and hot sauces

Not on the Program
- Ultimate Burrito (633 calories)
- Mexican Chicken Caesar Burrito (734 calories)
- Chicken Fiesta Salad (756 calories)
- Chicken Tostada Salad (990 calories)

EL TORITO

www.eltorito.com

Before eating here, reread the section on dining in Mexican restaurants (page 40). El Torito is pretty traditional, which means lots of fried food, lots of cheese, and lots of extra fat added to most (but not all) of the food.

Top Picks
- Chicken Soft Tacos
- Fresh Fish Tacos
- Chicken Breast or Fresh Fish Fajitas
- Sonora Burrito Lite
- Grilled Chicken Salad—Make sure they hold any fatty extras such as sour cream and guacamole.
- Rice
- Corn Tortilla
- Tortilla soup—If you can resist them, don't eat the fried tortilla strips that generally come with tortilla soup.

Not on the Program
- Macho Combo—Let's just say it's lots and lots of food.
- Chicken Flautas Rancheras
- Carne Asada Burrito
- Chile Relleno

FAZOLI'S

www.fazolis.com

If you know the drill for traditional Italian food, you'll fare okay here. Watch out for classic fat traps such as pastas Alfredo, cheesy pizzas, and those addictive garlic butter–brushed breadsticks they put on the table. Fazoli's also offers panini Italian sandwiches that are generally grilled or "pressed" in an iron. They're wonderful but best for a splurge since they generally incorporate cheese. (If you can get them to make a panino without cheese, then go for it.)

Top Picks
- Spaghetti with Marinara (420 calories; regular size 620 calories)
- Spaghetti with Meat Sauce (450 calories; regular size 670 calories)

TIP: The pastas here are served in both reduced and full-sized servings. As you can see by the numbers above, going for the smaller order will save you about 200 calories.

- Minestrone Soup (120 calories)
- Garden Salad with Reduced Calorie Italian Dressing (80 calories)
- Chicken Finger Salad with Reduced Calorie Italian Dressing (140 calories)

Not on the Program
- Submarino Club (1,100 calories)

- Spaghetti with Meatballs (regular size, 1,020 calories)
- Broccoli Lasagna (750 calories)
- Baked Chicken Alfredo (790 calories)

FUDDRUCKERS

www.fuddruckers.com

There's a lot on the menu here for people who like to eat "big." For those of us who like to eat in moderation, there are just a few selections. But sometimes it takes just one dish: I'm a big fan of the fish sandwich here (not available at all locations). One caveat: Beware the "specialty toppings," which can be high in calories.

Top Picks
- Grilled Fish Sandwich—Some Fuddruckers have this delicious sandwich (others have a fried fish sandwich, which, of course, is not on the program). It comes with a mayonnaise-based spread, but because the fish is so well seasoned, you don't need it.
- Portobello Mushroom Burger—A nice change of pace on a rather meat-heavy menu. Ask them to hold the cheese.
- Turkey, Garden, or Ostrich Burger
- Grilled Chicken Breast Sandwich
- Grilled Chicken Salad—Ask for the dressing on the side.
- Soup and Salad—As long as it's not a cream soup.

Not on the Program
- Southwest Burger
- The "Works" Crispy Chicken Sandwich
- Steakhouse Platters

GODFATHER'S PIZZA

Godfather's pretty much sticks to pizza with a few sandwiches. Stick to the basics here.

Top Picks
- Two slices of cheese pizza
- Salad bar—As always, watch the add-ons.

Not on the Program
- Combo Pizza—The calorie count per slice jumps about 100 calories when you go from plain cheese pizza to the combo, which has pepperoni, sausage, *and* beef.
- Super Specialty Pizzas
- Garlic Bread

HARDEE'S

www.hardeesrestaurants.com

Like most convenience eateries, Hardee's has its fair share of pitfalls. Fortunately, it has a few acceptable items and offers some foods in both smaller and larger sizes. Hardee's also serves breakfast, but I'd pass—there's really not much of a choice for the health-conscious diner.

Top Picks
- Chicken Slammer (278 calories)
- Grilled Chicken Sandwich (350 calories)
- Regular Roast Beef Sandwich (310 calories)

Not on the Program
- ½-pound Grilled Sourdough Burger (1,010 calories)
- ⅔-pound Monster Thickburger (1,201 calories)
- Fish Supreme Sandwich (520 calories)
- Big Chicken Filet Sandwich (716 calories)

IN-N-OUT BURGER

www.in-n-out.com

This family-owned chain gets kudos from fast-food aficionados for its high-quality made-to-order items. Yet in the end, In-N-Out still has a classic menu of hamburgers, fries, and shakes—and a very limited menu at that.

Top Picks

- Burger Without the Burger—This is a trick that many vegetarians use when they end up at In-N-Out. You can order a sandwich of lettuce, tomato, cheese, and grilled (or fresh) onions. You can even ask them to hold the cheese; they're very accommodating here. Ask for mustard and ketchup instead of the mayonnaise-based spread.
- Burger Without the Bun—If you like, they'll wrap your hamburger in lettuce leaves and hold the bun. Spartan, I know, but, hey, I told you it was slim pickin's!

TIP: Compare the calorie counts: regular hamburger off the menu, 390 calories; with mustard and ketchup instead of spread, 310 calories; with lettuce leaves instead of a bun, 240 calories.

Not on the Program

- Double-Double (670 calories)

INTERNATIONAL HOUSE OF PANCAKES (IHOP)

www.ihop.com

Pancakes are definitely a once-in-a-while food for people on the program, mostly because of all the syrup and butter people heap on top of them. It goes without saying that you should skip the butter, but also use a light hand with the syrup since those sugary calories add up and they really don't have a lot of nutrients. If you had eggs, at least you'd be getting some protein and vitamins. If you find yourself in IHOP for lunch or dinner, forgo the pancakes completely—there are several alternatives on the menu that are a lot healthier.

Top Picks
Breakfast
- Eggs and whole-wheat toast

TIP: If going to a pancake house and not having pancakes is out of the question for you, order *one* pancake on the side *instead of toast.*

- Crepe-Style International Pancakes—These are lighter than traditional pancakes. Order them without the sauce and butter and use a bit of syrup instead.
- Harvest Grain 'N Nut Pancakes—You'll probably get more calories than you need in this dish, but at least you'll also get some nutrient-rich oats, almonds, and walnuts.

Lunch and Dinner
- Breast of Chicken Sandwich with salad or soup
- Turkey Sandwich with salad or soup
- Grilled Chicken Breast

Not on the Program
Breakfast
- Breakfast Sampler—No one really needs eggs, bacon, ham, pork sausage, hash browns, and buttermilk pancakes all in one meal.
- Country Fried Steak and Eggs
- Country Omelette
- Pigs in Blankets

Lunch and Dinner
- Double BLT
- Hamburger Club
- Southwestern Chicken Fajita Salad
- Signature Sampler

JACK IN THE BOX
www.jackinthebox.com
Like some other big-name fast-food restaurants, Jack in the Box is making an effort to offer some more healthful choices, entering the "salad wars" with some enticing dishes; but in this case, you need to use caution.

Top Picks

- Chicken Fajita Pita (330 calories)—This is your number one choice here. It's relatively low in calories and not swimming in fat.
- Chicken Teriyaki Bowl (550 calories)—It's not your lowest-calorie option, but with only 3 grams of fat (less than 1 gram of it saturated), it's your leanest.
- Chipotle Chicken (390 calories)
- Hamburger (310 calories)—A plain old hamburger (and I do mean plain—don't put anything like cheese on it) is not your worst choice. It has 6 grams of saturated fat, which isn't much more than the chicken entrées have.
- Taco (170 calories)

Breakfast

- Breakfast Jack (310 calories)

Not on the Program

- Salads (610–830 calories)—Ultimately, I can't recommend these salads. On the one hand, they include some fresh, healthy ingredients. On the other hand, there are also many fatty extras added to them. The Asian Chicken Salad has wonton strips and a high-calorie dressing; the Southwest Chicken Salad has cheese and corn sticks tossed in; the Chicken Club Salad has cheese, bacon, and croutons, and a bacon dressing. If you are going to order one (the Asian is the best option), at least ask for Jack in the Box's Low-Calorie Italian Dressing.
- Bacon Ultimate Cheeseburger (1,120 calories)
- Jack's Spicy Chicken (650 calories)—Proving again that chicken sandwiches aren't always low in calories.
- Stuffed Jalapeños (230 calories/three)

Breakfast

- Everything but the Breakfast Jack

JAMBA JUICE

www.jambajuice.com

Though I haven't included many drink or coffee shops in this guide, I want you to get a sense of how many calories you're getting when you drink juice, and smoothies in particular. Smoothies (fruit and juices blended with ice to make a thick shakelike drink) are generally very nutritious, and they provide people who don't eat much produce with an easy way to increase their fruit—and sometimes vegetable—intake. Yet eating fruits and vegetables in their natural state is a healthier proposition since a lot of fiber, which both is filling and protects against disease, is lost in the juicing process. If you're going to drink juices and smoothies, keep in mind the calorie content and balance the rest of your meals and snacks accordingly.

Top Picks
- Orange/Carrot Juice (160 calories/16 ounces)
- Vibrant C
- Orange/Banana Juice (220 calories/16 ounces)

TIP: Go with a friend, order one smoothie or juice and ask for two cups. The servings are big to begin with, so you'll get a more reasonable portion if you split.

- Grin N' Carrot (250 calories)
- Honey Berry Bran (320 calories)
- Lemon Poppyseed Bundt (300 calories)

TIP: The calorie counts for the muffins here is actually very reasonable, and they are made with healthy oils.

Not on the Program
- Peanut Butter Moo'd (860 calories/24 ounces)
- Peenya Kowlada (650 calories/24 ounces)
- Kiwi Berry Burner (470 calories/24 ounces)

- Stawberries Wild (450 calories/24 ounces)
- Sourdough Parmesan Pretzel (460 calories)

JOHNNY ROCKETS

www.johnnyrockets.com

As you might expect from a place that subtitles itself "The Original Hamburger," here burgers are king. The good news is that they'll substitute a lean ground turkey patty for the traditional red-meat burger. There are also a few (and just a few) other acceptable options on the menu.

Top Picks

- The Original with a turkey patty—This is a simple burger with lettuce, tomato, onion, relish, pickle, mustard, and mayonnaise. Ask them to leave the mayo off your order.
- Streamliner Vegetarian burger—A Boca burger with the works, but hold the mayo.

TIP: Adding grilled onions and mushrooms to your burgers is a good way to get more vegetables on your plate.

- Grilled Breast of Chicken Sandwich
- Chicken Club Sandwich—It's made with fried or grilled chicken. You know which one to ask for. And hold the bacon and cheese.

Not on the Program

- St. Louis Burger
- Chili Size
- Chicken Club Sandwich

KENNY ROGERS ROASTERS ★

www.nathansfamous.com

If you're partial to fast-food chicken, this is a great alternative to a fried chicken restaurant.

The chicken (and turkey) here is wood fire–roasted, so it has a lot of flavor but not much fat. Remember, though, that much of the fat in chicken and turkey is contained in the skin, so it's a good idea to remove it before eating. Kenny Rogers also offers some nutritious vegetable side dishes. Some of them include butter, so keep in mind the top picks below.

Top Picks
- Original Grilled Chicken Breast Sandwich—Hold the mayo.
- White Meat Turkey on a roll—Likewise.
- Grilled Vegetable Pita or Wrap
- Roasted Chicken Strip Salad
- Chicken Noodle Soup
- Wood-Roasted Turkey Breast
- Grilled Chicken Breast Fillet

TIP: Forgo the sandwich and just order turkey or chicken and a few vegetable sides.

- Tomato-Cucumber and Onion Salad
- Herb Italian Green Beans
- Peas and Carrots
- Butternut Squash
- Baked Sweet Potato
- Grilled Vegetables

Not on the Program
- Krispy Chicken Tender on a roll
- Caesar Salad
- Honey-Bourbon Barbecue Ribs
- Garlic Potatoes
- Sour Cream and Dill Pasta Salad
- Corn Niblets
- Creamy Parmesan Spinach
- Chicken Pot Pie

KENTUCKY FRIED CHICKEN

KFC has a page on its Web site devoted to animal welfare and the company's efforts to promote the humane treatment of chickens. That's commendable, but I wish KFC would do something more to promote *human* welfare. Though it has a few healthier options, it really would be doing people a service if it added a few more.

Top Picks
- Tender Roast Sandwich without sauce (277 calories)
- Honey BBQ Flavored Sandwich (310 calories)
- Corn on the Cob (150 calories)
- BBQ Baked Beans (190 calories)
- Green Beans (45 calories)
- Means Greens (70 calories)

Not on the Program
- Everything else

KOO KOO ROO ★

www.kookooroo.com

If you need proof that fast food doesn't have to be a greasy heart attack in a sack, this chain is it. Not only does it offer chicken without the skin, but it has a long list of vegetables that are cooked without any (or with very little) added fat. This is the kind of place you can feel comfortable dining at on a regular basis.

Top Picks
- Original Skinless Flame-Broiled Chicken, Original Breast (155 calories) or Original Breast and Wing (212 calories)
- Turkey Breast Sandwich with Lite Mayo (538 calories)
- ¼ pound Sliced White Turkey Meat (153 calories)

- Koo Koo Roo House Salad (164 calories without dressing)
- Turkey Dumpling Soup (166 calories)
- Ten Vegetable Soup (121 calories)
- Chicken Chili (98 calories)
- All of the hot side dishes except those noted below

TIP: You can make a nice meal on the vegetable side dishes alone: a plate of black beans, asparagus, butternut squash, and cracked wheat rice, for example.

- Lentil salad (176 calories)
- Tangy Tomato Salad (46 calories)

Not on the Program
- Chicken Caesar Sandwich
- Chicken Tostada Bowl with Cilantro Ranch Dressing
- Any of the wraps
- Turkey Pot Pie

KRYSTAL

www.krystalco.com

Krystal is your classic hamburger, hot dog, Coke, and fries type of place, which doesn't really make it *our* kind of place. Still, if you eat on the smaller side of its spectrum, a meal here won't do too much damage.

Top Picks
- Krystal Burger (160 calories)—A better choice than the Krystal Chik, which is "crispy," another word for fried (240 calories).
- Krystal Chili (200 calories)
- Plain Pup (170 calories)

Not on the Program
- Double Cheese Krystal (310 calories)
- Corn Pup (260 calories)

LA SALSA

Like most Mexican restaurants, La Salsa has many dishes that sound safe but which are actually very high in calories. Still, you can do well here if you keep your meal simple and stay away from dishes that come with sauce or have *grande*—Spanish for "large"—in their title.

Top Picks
- Sonoran Mahi Mahi Taco (200 calories)
- Mexico City Chicken Taco (210 calories)
- Mexico City Steak Taco (220 calories)
- Sonoran Mahi Mahi Burrito (540 calories)
- Rice (130 calories)
- Beans (240 calories)

Not on the Program
- Baja-Style Shrimp and Fish Tacos—Individually these don't have more calories than the Sonoran Mahi Mahi Burrito (the shrimp has 450, the fish 370). However, tacos are small, and if you eat two or more of them, the calories add up.
- All Burritos except the Sonoran
- Quesadillas
- Any Platters
- All salads, especially the Taco Salad (42 grams of fat!)

LITTLE CAESARS

www.littlecaesars.com

A slice is a slice is a slice? Not really. There are a few things that account for the difference in calories among slices of pizza. The most obvious factor, of course, is the topping. Second is the thickness of the crust. At Little Caesars, the Deep Dish pizza and regular-crust pizza are more fattening than a thin-crust pizza. But the size of the *entire* pizza also matters. Fourteen-inch pies are cut into larger pieces than twelve-inch pies are. And when you buy pizza that's sold by the slice, there are almost twice as many calories as in a slice from a twelve-inch pie. So really eyeball the pizza slice you're selecting. A bigger slice will make *you* bigger.

Top Picks
- Cheese slice from a twelve-inch thin-crust pie (141 calories)
- Tossed Side Salad with Fat Free Italian (146 calories)

Not on the Program
- Slice of Deep Dish pepperoni pizza (312 calories)
- Cold Sandwiches (600 to 720 calories)

LONG JOHN SILVER'S

www.ljsilvers.com
Just about everything here is fried, so your choices are very limited.

Top Picks
- Chicken Sandwich
- Corn Cobette
- Rice

Not on the Program
- Battered Fish, Shrimp, Clams, or Chicken
- Ultimate Fish Sandwich

MANHATTAN BAGEL

www.manhattanbagel.com
Bagels, of course, are this restaurant's bread and butter. It does, however, also offer sandwiches on "bakery breads," and I'd watch out for these: they often contain cheese, and tend to be even higher in calories than bagels. Stick to the basics here.

Top Picks
- Bagel with reduced-fat cream cheese
- Turkey sandwich with lettuce, cucumbers, tomato, and mustard (or salsa) on a bagel—This isn't on the menu, but Manhattan Bagel has all of the fixings—it just generally teams it with cheese or something like a Caesar dressing.
- Times Square, hold the Swiss—A ham sandwich with Dijon mustard.

Not on the Program
- Sandwiches on Bakery Breads
- Ellis Island—A bagel sandwich with pastrami and cheese.

MAZZIO'S

www.mazzios.com

The menu at Mazzio's is straightforward and limited. Besides pizza, it also has a selection of sandwiches and pasta—a better choice if you're willing to forgo a few slices.

Top Picks
- Turkey sandwich
- Spaghetti with Marinara
- Salad bar
- Cheese pizza with vegetable toppings (ask for half the cheese)

Not on the Program
- Three Pounder or Cheese Extreme pizzas
- Calzone Ring
- Chicken Fried Chicken Alfredo

MCDONALD'S

www.mcdonalds.com

McDonald's has a newfound commitment to providing patrons with healthier options. Some of the changes—such as the addition of premium salads to its offerings—are apparent. Others—such as encouraging meat and poultry producers to use fewer antibiotics—don't show up on the menu but are also important in promoting our well-being.

Top Picks

- Grilled Chicken Caesar Salad (300 calories)—Order it with Newman's Own Light Balsamic Vinaigrette (40 calories/1½ ounces).

TIP: I find that I don't even need to use a whole packet of dressing. Try sampling your salad with less than the 1½ ounces before you add the whole amount.

- Grilled Chicken Bacon Ranch Salad (360 calories)—Ditto.
- Grilled Chicken California Cobb Salad (370 calories)—Again, ordering the right dressing is key.

TIP: All the salads are also available without chicken, good to know if you've had enough protein for the day or are a vegetarian.

- Chicken McGrill (400 calories)—This has slightly less fat than the Grilled Chicken Flatbread and the McChicken.

Breakfast

- Scrambled eggs (160 calories)
- English muffin (150 calories)

Not on the Program

- Double Quarter Pounder with Cheese (760 calories)
- Chicken McNuggets (510 calories/ten pieces)—The problem is not so much the calories as the fat they're fried in.
- Big N' Tasty with Cheese (580 calories)

Breakfast
- Big Breakfast (710 calories)
- Spanish Omelette Bagel (710 calories)

MIAMI SUBS

www.miamisubs.com

This sub shop also has some Greek items on the menu, not something you ordinarily see in a fast-food restaurant. Bear in mind that subs are almost always high in calories. Since salads are available here, you might consider having half a sub (take the other half home or share) and a side salad.

Top Picks
- Chicken Pita (392 calories)
- Cheesesteak Original (409 calories)—It defies conventional logic, but the simple cheese steaks here are less caloric and have less total and saturated fat then the subs.
- Ham and Cheese Sub (451 calories)—Hold the cheese for fewer calories.
- Turkey Sub (483 calories)—Hold the mayo to slim it down.
- Garden Salad (309 calories)
- Greek Salad (284 calories)
- Side Greek Salad (78 calories)

Not on the Program
- Deluxe Bacon Cheeseburger (919 calories)
- Gyros Platter (1,420 calories)
- Chicken Philly Cheesesteak Classic (551 calories)

MIMI'S CAFE ★

www.mimiscafe.com

The offerings at Mimi's range from the seriously indulgent to rarefied (but much appreciated) health-conscious entrées. Everything is also made to order, so this is the kind of place where you can not only ask them to skip the mayo, they encourage you to do so. The restaurant's Web site even provides ordering tips.

Top Picks
Lunch and Dinner
- Turkey Sandwich—Request fruit on the side and no mayo. You may need only a half sandwich: they're pretty big.
- Chicken and Fruit—If you ask, they'll bring you nonfat dressing.
- Spaghettini with Tomatoes and Basil
- Shrimp Spaghettini
- Roasted Turkey Breast—Swap sliced tomatoes for the potatoes.
- Broiled Halibut Steak—Ditto.
- Broiled King Salmon
- Soup—Of the noncream variety, naturally.
- Salads—Most of the salads here are garnished with calorie-dense extras such as wonton noodles and bleu cheese. If you can't resist, at least they come in petite sizes, but better yet, order a big green salad and Mimi's Nonfat Dressing.
- BBQ Turkey Burger—Ask for fruit or soup instead of fries.
- Chicken Burger
- Honey Mandarin Chicken—A boneless breast; take off the skin.

Breakfast
- Eggs to Egg Beaters—They'll gladly substitute tomatoes for potatoes.
- Egg Beaters Fitness Omelette—Made with lots of veggies and served with dry wheat toast.
- Oatmeal
- Cheerios

Not on the Program
- French Quarter—A gigantic hamburger with every fatty fixing you can think of.

- Five-Way Grilled Cheese—Need I say more?
- J.B.'s 14 ounces Rib Eye
- Pasta Jambalaya
- Penne with Chicken, Feta, and Pine Nuts

Breakfast
- Eggs Houssard
- Chipotle Breakfast Burrito
- Mimi's Thick Egg French Toast

NATHAN'S FAMOUS

www.nathansfamous.com

For those of you who associate it with Coney Island, Nathan's may be a great place to go for nostalgia, but it's not the ideal spot for healthy eating—you know you're in trouble when a hot dog is one of the lowest-fat items on the menu! Think of it as a splurge destination, not for run-of-the-mill meals.

Top Picks
- Nathan's Famous Hot Dog
- Chargrilled Chicken Sandwich

Not on the Program
- Super Burger
- Cheesesteak Supreme
- Hot Dog Nuggets

OLIVE GARDEN ★

Many of the classic rules for dining at Italian restaurants (see page 38) apply here: Watch out for anything called "Alfredo" or "Parmigiana," think beyond pasta, explore the soup options, and so on. But the Olive Garden also makes it a little easier on you by creating what it calls "Garden Fare." Stick to those dishes, and you'll do fine.

Top Picks
These are all from the Garden Fare menu.

- Linguine alla Marinara (280 calories/lunch portion; 450 calories/dinner portion)
- Chicken Giardino (350 calories/lunch portion; 460 calories/dinner portion)
- Capellini Pomodoro (350 calories/lunch portion; 560 calories/dinner portion)
- Shrimp Primavera (490 calories/lunch portion; 730 calories/dinner portion)
- Minestrone Soup (100 calories)

From the regular menu:

- Swordfish Piccata—As long as they'll serve it without the sauce.

Not on the Program
- Cucina Classica (except those entrées mentioned above)—These tend to have lots of cheese or creamy sauces.
- Cannelloni al Forno—Lots of meat and cream.
- Tortelloni de Fizzano—Lots of meat, cheese, and cream.

1 POTATO 2 ★

Although its name would lead you to believe that this eatery serves nothing but potatoes, it actually has quite a varied menu. There's a little bit of everything here, and it's made an effort to include quite a few healthy dishes.

Top Picks
- Baked Potato—These come all dressed up with cheese and other toppings. See if you can get one plain, then use a little Low Fat Ranch dressing to jazz it up.
- ½ Sandwich & Cup o' Soup—Your best sandwich pick? See below.

- Grilled Chicken Pita Sandwich—Ask for the sauce on the side or skip it altogether.
- Grilled Chicken Sandwich—This isn't exactly on the menu, but another sandwich—Cajun Chicken Club—includes a grilled breast, so I'm sure they will make you a plain sandwich if you ask.

TIP: You can order a side of steamed vegetables instead of fries.

- Chicken Breast Dinner
- Lemon Pepper Cod—Ask them not to broil it in butter as they usually do.

Not on the Program
- Baked Potato with Chili and Cheddar
- Reuben Sandwich
- Turkey Croissant Sandwich
- Potato Pancakes
- Chicken Fettuccini

OUTBACK STEAKHOUSE

www.outbacksteakhouse.com

The Australian theme of this restaurant makes it tempting to adopt an Australian devil-may-care attitude toward eating, yet try not to get too caught up in the moment. Besides, the menu has quite a bit more to offer than colossal deep-fried shrimp, giant steaks, and the Bloomin' Onion— a fried concoction that the watchdog group Center for Science in the Public Interest estimates has 1,690 calories and 116 grams of fat! Stay the course by choosing mostly grilled items.

Top Picks
- Soup 'N Salad—As long as the soup isn't cream-based.
- Grilled Chicken Breast—This isn't exactly on the menu; however, a dish called Sweet Chook o' Mine is made with a grilled chicken breast (plus

cheese and bacon), so you should be able to get the chicken plain.

- Botany Bay Fish o' the Day
- North Atlantic Salmon
- Chicken and Veggie Griller
- Shrimp and Veggie Griller
- Victoria's Filet—This is a 9-ounce steak and a much better choice than the other, bigger cuts.

Not on the Program
- Queensland Salad—It has chicken, but also cheese, bacon, and egg.
- All steaks except if you're sharing or order the one mentioned above.
- Alice Springs Chicken—Chicken covered in saturated fat.

PANDA EXPRESS

www.pandaexpress.com

Because Panda Express, a fast-food Chinese eatery, doesn't cook food to order, you won't be able to make some of the requests you can make at other Chinese restaurants. The key here is to stick with the regular versus the large portion sizes and, if you choose a combination plate, to get only one or two entrées. Also, of course, stay away from anything deep-fried.

Top Picks
- Chicken with Mushrooms
- Fresh Mixed Vegetables
- Mandarin Chicken Bowl
- Beef with Broccoli
- Steamed Rice

Not on the Program
- Chicken Egg Roll
- Vegetable Fried Rice
- Spicy Chicken with Peanuts—While peanuts are

relatively healthy (unless you're allergic), they drive up the calorie count in this dish.

PAPA JOHN'S PIZZA

www.papajohns.com

Pizza is almost exclusively the name of the game here—it doesn't even offer salads (at least not at the branches I checked out) so use your pie-ordering smarts, such as remembering to ask for half the cheese. Note that it offers thin-crust pizza here, which will help you save quite a few calories.

Top Picks

- Thin Crust Cheese or Garden Special Pizza—The thin crust has about 50 fewer calories per slice than the original crust.

Not on the Program

- All the Meat Pizzas
- Cheese Sticks

PERKINS RESTAURANT & BAKERY ★

www.perkinsrestaurants.com

Like any country-style restaurant, Perkins has its share of overly hearty meals. Yet it's quite possible to find not just one or two but several different healthy meal choices here. What I like about this place is that it gives you a choice right on the menu: Do you, for instance, want your grouper grilled or fried? It's nice not to feel that you have to special-order every time you walk into an establishment.

Top Picks

- Grilled Apricot Teriyaki Salmon—The sides you're offered include steamed broccoli and baked potatoes, both good choices.
- Grilled Grouper or Atlantic Cod

- Teriyaki Chicken Grille
- Create Your Own Pasta—You can choose among sauces and toppings. I'd go for the marinara with a topping of portobello mushrooms and/or chicken breast.
- Plain Chicken Sandwich—This isn't actually on the menu—the chicken sandwiches that are have bacon or cheese and bacon—but it should be no problem to have them pare it down to the basics for you.
- Garden Salad with Fat-Free Italian dressing
- Perkins Famous Chicken Noodle Soup

Breakfast
- Two Egg Combo
- Egg Beaters Scramble
- Oatmeal
- Cold Cereal
- Fruit

Not on the Program
- Rodeo Burger
- Parmesan Grillers—Giant sandwiches with lots of cheese.
- Perkins Country Fried Steak
- Perkins Baskets—Essentially fried fish (or chicken) and chips.

Breakfast
- Tremendous Twelve—A mess of eggs, pancakes, hash browns, and bacon.
- Deli-Ham and Lots-A-Cheese Omelette
- Cinnamon Roll French Toast
- Mammoth Muffin

PETER PIPER PIZZA

www.peterpiperpizza.com
This is a classic pizza place with the classic fat traps. It offers salads so you can opt out of the pizza if you desire; just go easy on the dressing.

The Peter Piper I tried didn't offer low-fat or nonfat dressings, so bring your own. Otherwise you're at their mercy.

Top Picks
- Two small slices of original crust pizza (plain or California Classic, which is piled high with vegetables)—This is a lower-calorie option than the personal pizza.
- Salad

Not on the Program
- Bacon Double Cheeseburger pizza
- The Werx pizza

PF CHANG'S CHINA BISTRO

This upscale Chinese food chain serves its food relatively "clean"—that is, not drowning in greasy sauces. It even has some acceptable appetizers, a rarity for *any* restaurant, let alone a Chinese one. Still, use caution when ordering here, since even lightly sauced Chinese food has lots of hidden fat and calories.

Top Picks
Appetizers:
- Chang's Chicken in Soothing Lettuce Wraps or Chang's Vegetarian Lettuce Wraps—This appetizer is served in a lettuce leaf instead of a doughy wrapper.
- Shrimp or Vegetable Dumplings, steamed
- Seared Ahi Tuna
- Shanghai Cucumbers

Soups:
- Hot and Sour Soup
- Wonton Soup

Entrées:
- Steamed Fish of the Day

- Oolong Marinated Sea Bass
- Cantonese Scallops or Shrimp
- Ginger Chicken with Broccoli
- Mango Chicken

Vegetables:
- Sichuan-Style Long Beans or Asparagus
- Buddha's Feast

Not on the Program
Appetizers:
- Pan-Fried Dumplings
- Crab Wontons

Entrées:
- Sweet and Sour Pork
- Crispy Honey Shrimp
- Orange Peel Beef

Vegetables and Noodles:
- Stir-Fried Spicy Eggplant—Eggplant soaks up oil like a sponge.
- Double Pan-Fried Noodles

PICK UP STIX

www.pickupstix.com

Pick Up Stix might not be exactly what you'd call a fast-food restaurant, but it fixes food fast, and I think that if you order wisely, you'll end up with a much healthier meal than even your typical fast-food grilled chicken sandwich.

Top Picks
- Wonton Soup
- Hot and Sour Soup
- Mandarin Garden Side Salad with Fat-Free Spicy Lime Cilantro dressing
- Vegetable Sauté
- Shrimp with Vegetables
- Chicken with Vegetables

Not on the Program
- Fried Rice
- Chow Mein
- Mongolian Beef
- Sweet and Sour Chicken

PIZZA HUT

www.pizzahut.com

Pizza Hut offers so many different types of crusts, it can make your head spin. While I suppose that's nice from a gastronomic point of a view, from a health point of view it can be confusing—and believe me, there's a big difference among the different crusts. The information below will assist you, but also use your eyes: if it looks bulky, it probably will make *you* bulky, too.

Top Picks
- Thin 'N Crispy Pizza (200 calories/slice)
- Hand Tossed Pizza (240 calories/slice)
- Spaghetti with Marinara (490 calories)—While not necessarily less caloric than a couple of slices of pizza, this dish has far less saturated fat.
- Salad with Reduced Calorie Creamy Cucumber Dressing (30 calories for the dressing)

Not on the Program
- Personal Pan Pizza (630 calories each)
- Stuffed Crust Gold Pizza (440 calories/slice)
- The Big New Yorker Pizza (410 calories/slice)
- The Chicago Dish Pizza (390 calories/slice)
- Stuffed Crust Pizza (360 calories/slice)
- Pan Pizza (290 calories/slice)

PIZZERIA UNO CHICAGO GRILL

www.pizzeriauno.com

Pizza is generally what you think of when you think of Unos; however, this restaurant has a lot more to offer. Which is a good thing: its specialty, deep-dish pizza, is definitely not on the program. Do a good search of the menu here, and you'll find some healthy options.

Top Picks
- House Salad with Grilled Shrimp, Chicken, or Salmon—Fat-free dressings are available.
- Grilled Shrimp and Roasted Vegetable Salad
- Thin Crust Cheese and Tomato Pizza or with vegetables
- Teriyaki Salmon
- Teriyaki Chicken
- Grilled Chicken Breast Sandwich
- Veggie Burger

Not on the Program
- French Onion Soup
- Cream of Broccoli Soup
- 11-pound New York Strip Steak
- Deep Dish Pizza
- Lobster and Shrimp Pie
- Fish Sandwich

POPEYES

www.popeyes.com

This restaurant may have the same name as the legendary cartoon character, but you won't find his favorite food (spinach) here. Popeyes really isn't the type of place you should go if you're trying to stay on the program because just about everything is fried. However, if you do find yourself in one, go for the side dishes.

Top Picks
- Red Beans and Rice
- Corn on the Cob

Not on the Program
- Fried Chicken, Shrimp, and Catfish

QUIZNOS SUB ★

www.quiznos.com

Submarine sandwiches are by nature hefty, and where there's heft, there are calories. Quiznos has done us the favor of creating a few sandwiches that each has fewer than 7 grams of fat. Remember these choices, and you'll always be able to order wisely here.

Top Picks

- Small Turkey Lite on Wheat Bread (334 calories)
- Small Honey Bourbon Chicken on Wheat Bread (359 calories)
- Small Sierra Smoked Turkey on Italian Ciabatta Bread (350 calories)
- Deli Oven Roasted Turkey—Hold the mayo.
- Side Garden Salad
- Chicken Noodle Soup

Not on the Program

- Signature Subs, especially the Classic Italian

RALLY'S

Rally's specializes in hamburgers and has a pretty small menu. If you can't resist the hamburgers, get a small one.

Top Picks

- Honey Grilled Chicken Sandwich—It comes with a honey mustard sauce rather than your typical mayo-based spread.
- Small Rallyburger

Not on the Program

- Big Buford—A double burger, twice as much as you need.
- Double BBQ Bacon Cheeseburger
- Beer Battered Onions

RAX ★

At some restaurants, what you see on the menu is what you get. At Rax, they're open to shaving some of the mayo and oil off the sandwiches, potatoes, and salads to make you a healthier meal. All you have to do is ask.

Top Picks

- Deli Turkey Sandwich (233 calories)—Keep it simple.
- Grilled Chicken Sandwich (283 calories)—Hold the mayo.
- Jr. Deluxe Roast Beef Sandwich (215 calories)—A good choice if you hold the fatty fixings.
- Baked Potato, plain (207 calories)
- Grilled Chicken Salad with Fat Free dressing (190 calories)
- Salad bar, when available
- Cream of Broccoli Soup (95 calories)—An exception to the "no cream soups" rule.
- Chicken Noodle Soup (113 calories)
- Chili (158 calories)

Not on the Program

- Turkey Bacon Club Sandwich (680 calories)
- BBC Sandwich (716 calories)

RED LOBSTER SEAFOOD RESTAURANTS ★

www.redlobster.com

You can feel pretty confident when you walk into a seafood restaurant that you're going to find something that won't knock you off the program. That holds true for Red Lobster, though the chain also has its fair share of fried dishes on the menu. Two words to keep in mind here: broiled and grilled!

Top Picks

- Jumbo Shrimp Cocktail

- Fresh fish, broiled or grilled—The options range from flounder to mahi mahi.
- Broiled seafood platter
- Dockside Shrimp and Chicken
- Lobster, steamed—But only if you're willing to eat it without butter.
- Teriyaki chicken

Not on the Program
- Boardwalk Popcorn Shrimp
- Admiral's Feast—Apparently the admiral liked his fried.
- Cajun Shrimp Linguini

RED ROBIN GOURMET BURGERS

www.redrobin.com

Red Robin is essentially a burger joint that also serves a mix of Mexican- and Asian-influenced dishes. It offers an admirable list of alternatives to the typical burger; however, you also have to be careful to give specific directions when you order—they tend to put cheese on everything here.

Top Picks
- Grilled Turkey Burger—Hold the mayo.
- Amazing Veggie Burger
- Boca Burger
- Lauren's Portobello Burger—A big mushroom sandwich. Don't forget to tell them to hold the cheese and mayo. When you buy this dish, Red Robin donates 50 cents to a children's charity. Nice touch.

TIP: At this and other restaurants with a long list of burgers on the menu, it pays to read about all of the toppings even if you won't be ordering a beef patty. Sometimes the healthier burgers, such as vegetarian and turkey patties, come just with lettuce and tomato. But if you see that the restaurant also offers vegetable toppings on the meat burgers—grilled onions, mushrooms, or salsa, for instance—there's a good chance you can get it on your healthier burger, too.

- Chicken Burger—All the chicken burgers are gunked up with something (cheese, guacamole, fried onions). Ask for just a plain grilled chicken burger with vegetable toppings.
- Soup and Salad Combo—The tortilla soup (hold the cheese and sour cream) is your best bet with Lo-Cal Ranch or Italian on the salad.

Not on the Program
- Monster Burger
- Salads other than dinner salad
- Seafood Pasta

ROMANO'S MACARONI GRILL
www.macaronigrill.com

Although this is a fairly large chain, it hasn't created any special dishes for people watching their weight or the condition of their arteries. That said, it seems to be open to special requests, which can go a long way toward ensuring that you end up with a healthy meal.

Top Picks
- Grilled Salmon
- Capellini Pomodoro, plain or with chicken or shrimp—Served with a straightforward tomato sauce.
- Penne Arrabbiata, plain or with chicken or shrimp—Likewise, but with spice.
- Create your own pasta—This is a great option. You can stack your pasta with veggies and ask for the leanest sauce or just a touch of olive oil.

Not on the Program
- Antipasti—You can't really go right with any of these high-calorie appetizers.

- Any of the Italian Favorites
- Chicken, Salmon, or Veal Scaloppine

ROUND TABLE PIZZA

www.roundtablepizza.com

From the pizzas to the sandwiches to the salads, just about everything here has cheese on it. That means you can't be haphazard about ordering or take it for granted that a "veggie" sandwich ordered straight from the menu will be a good choice. Ask for less cheese on your pizza and no cheese in your salads and sandwiches.

Top Picks

- Turkey, Chicken, or Ham Sandwich—These aren't on the menu, but Turkey and Chicken Club Sandwiches are. Get them to make you a simple sandwich without the cheese, bacon, or Creamy Ranch Sauce.
- Veggie Sandwich—Ditto, without cheese or sauce.
- Garden Salad
- Personal Thin Crust Cheese, Gourmet Veggie, or Chicken and Garlic Gourmet Pizza

Not on the Program

- Caesar Salad
- King Arthur Supreme Pizza
- Montague's All Meat Marvel Pizza

ROY ROGERS

The pickings here are slim for those eschewing saturated and trans fats, but you can make a meal out of the few lower-calorie offerings. Try the side dishes. Roy Rogers also serves breakfast, but I don't recommend it.

Top Picks

- Grilled Chicken Salad

- Garden Salad
- Grilled Chicken Breast Sandwich
- Jr. Hamburger
- Plain Baked Potato
- Corn
- Green Beans
- Chicken Soup

Not on the Program
- Ground Sirloin Steak
- Chicken Nuggets
- Macaroni and Cheese

RUBIO'S FRESH MEXICAN GRILL ★

www.rubios.com

Sombreros off to Rubio's for creating what they call a "HealthMex" menu. These entrées are versions of items on the regular menu, but slimmed down in fat and calories. Authentic Mexican food can be essentially healthy, and Rubio's takes it back to its basic goodness. Why don't I recommend something like the Fish Taco Especial, even though it has fewer calories than the HealthMex Burrito? Because most people eat at least two tacos, which amounts to more calories than are in the burrito.

Top Picks
- HealthMex Chicken or Fish Taco (170 calories/180 calories)
- HealthMex Grilled Fish Burrito (550 calories)
- HealthMex Veggie Burrito (470 calories)
- Grilled Chicken Chopped Salad (540 calories)
- Rice (110 calories)
- Beans (220–250 calories)

TIP: There's a great salsa bar here, which gives you lots of options for adding flavor to your food with little caloric impact.

Not on the Program
- Fish Taco Especial (370 calories)
- Quesadillas (980–1,140 calories)
- Carne Asada Especial Burrito (1,020 calories)

SCHLOTZSKY'S DELI ★

www.schlotzskys.com

Deli is not a word I usually associate with healthy food, but Schlotzsky's turns that notion on its head. It has a wide selection of choices, and many of them are right in line with the program. It's heartening to see that it seems to have gone out of its way to please all kinds of eaters. One of the things I like about its menu is that the sandwiches come in small, regular, and large sizes. It's a nice acknowledgment that not everyone wants to eat supersize portions.

Top Picks
Salads:
- Fresh Fruit Salad (123 calories)
- Albacore Tuna Salad (218 calories)—I don't generally recommend tuna salad, but Schlotzsky's makes its with olive oil, not mayonnaise.
- California Pasta Salad (58 calories)
- Garden Salad with Light Spicy Ranch or Light Italian Dressing (188 calories/138 calories)

Soups:
- Minestrone (89 calories)
- Old-Fashioned Chicken Noodle (122 calories)
- Ravioli (111 calories)
- Red Beans and Rice (167 calories)
- Vegetarian Vegetable (138 calories)

Sandwiches:
- Chicken Breast, small (337 calories)
- Smoked Turkey Breast, small (335 calories)
- The Vegetarian, small (324 calories)
- Albacore Tuna, small (334 calories)—The tuna in

this sandwich is made with Fat Free Spicy Ranch Dressing.
- Tuscan Turkey, small (327 calories)
- Dijon Chicken, small (329 calories)
- Pesto Chicken, small (346 calories)
- Zesty Albacore Tuna Wrap (311 calories)

TIP: You get a pretty wide selection of bread here. Wheat is your best choice, followed by sourdough and dark rye. Forgo the jalapeño cheese and rosemary Parmesan varieties.

Not on the Program
- Chicken and Pesto Pasta Salad (454 calories)
- Tuscan Tomato Basil Soup (320 calories)—This soup has 29 grams of fat!
- Chicken with Wild Rice (360 calories)—19 grams of fat!
- Pizza (upward of 524 calories)
- Fiesta Chicken Sandwich, large (1,598 calories)
- Pastrami and Swiss Sandwich, large (1,748 calories)
- Philly Sandwich, large (1,615 calories)
- Turkey Guacamole Sandwich, large (1,262 calories)

SHAKEY'S

www.shakeys.com

Whenever a pizza place offers something other than pizza, I consider it a good thing. Not that you should give up pizza entirely, but if you frequently end up in pizza parlors and all you eat is pizza, you're eventually going to notice it around your waist. Shakey's doesn't offer a lot of other dishes beside pizza that I would recommend, but there a few.

Top Picks
- Salad Bar
- Spaghetti—Without the garlic bread.
- Thin Crust Pizza with vegetables

Not on the Program

- Family Meal Deals—These are pizzas with the addition of things such as fried chicken or fried fish.
- Mojo Potatoes

SHONEY'S

www.shoneys.com

Although it's a good old-fashioned restaurant that's been around for years, Shoney's has created some dishes that address our modern concerns about high cholesterol and excess calories. One thing to watch out for here is the buffet. I recommend sticking to the regular menu.

Top Picks

- Chicken or Shrimp Stir-Fry—Skip the accompanying egg roll.
- Charbroiled Chicken Breast
- Grilled Catfish, Shrimp, or Cod
- House soup (noncreamy) and salad with vegetable buffet

Not on the Program

- Smothered Chicken
- Burgers
- Steaks
- Original Slim Jim—Smothered with cheese, it's not as slim as its name would have you believe.
- The Buffet (except for the vegetable buffet offered as a side)

SIZZLER ★

www.sizzler.com

The nice thing about Sizzler is that, even though it's known for its reasonably priced steaks, you know you can always get lean chicken and seafood entrées as well. The dishes are all fairly simple, so you don't have to try to read between the lines of the menu to figure out what you're getting. And, of course, everything is made to order, so don't be shy about asking them to go easy (or eliminate) oil and butter.

Top Picks
- Lemon Herb Chicken—A skinless breast, but ask for the sauce on the side.
- Hibachi chicken
- Grilled Salmon
- Salad Bar—Only if you feel you can rein in your impulse to load up on the appetizers and dessert included in this meal.
- Grilled Cajun Chicken—Hold the cheese and mayo.
- Sizzlin' Grilled Shrimp Skewers

Not on the Program
- Mega Bacon Burger
- Fisherman's Platter—Lots o' fried fish.
- Crispy Chicken with Fettuccine Alfredo

SKIPPERS ★

The motto at this seafood house is "Eat More Fish!" That's certainly possible because it makes fish the right way—grilled. Of course, there's also lots of battered and fried seafood for grease-loving diehards, but happily there's a lot here for you, too.

Top Picks
- Grilled Cod Fillet (102 calories)
- Grilled Halibut Fillet (157 calories)
- Grilled Chicken Breast (125 calories)
- Grilled Chicken Teriyaki Breast (215 calories)
- Grilled Salmon Fillet (239 calories)
- Chowder (150 calories)
- Baked Potato (218 calories)

Not on the Program
- Battered Salmon (190 calories)
- Breaded Clam Strips (450 calories)
- Grilled Chicken Caesar Salad (650 calories)

SONIC DRIVE-IN

www.sonicdrivein.com

The nostalgic part of me loves the idea of a drive-in; the contemporary part of me wishes that Sonic had more healthy options. This is a place it's probably better to patronize when you're allowing yourself to splurge than for an everyday, nutrition-conscious meal. That said, you'll find a few items on the menu that you can enjoy and stay on the program.

Top Picks
- Grilled Chicken Wrap without Ranch Dressing (393 calories)—The dressing adds another 150 calories.
- Grilled Cheese (282 calories)—Ordinarily I wouldn't put this on the Top Picks list, but it's actually one of the lowest-calorie dishes on the menu and has only a little more saturated fat than the Grilled Chicken Sandwich.
- Grilled Chicken Sandwich (343 calories)

Not on the Program
- Fritos Chili Cheese Wrap
- Country Fried Steak Toaster Sandwich
- Burgers

SOUPLANTATION AND SWEET TOMATOES ★

www.souplantation.com

It's not hard to eat healthfully here: The buffet (there's more than a hundred feet of salad bar) is jam-packed with fresh, nutritious choices, and the restaurant has gone out of its way to offer many reduced-calorie items. This is the one time I don't mind the buffet concept. Nonetheless, at a place like this you really have to exercise self-control. While there are many, many good selections on the salad bar, you can also get yourself into trouble by heaping too much of the wrong foods on your plate. The best strategy is to go heavy on all the plain vegetables, then use a light touch when adding extras such as dressings, nuts, seeds, and croutons. Also go easy on the prepared dishes and pretossed salads that are offered here, too. Many of them are low in calories and fat, but if you eat large portions (always a danger at a buffet), you'll end up with a lot more calories than you bargained for.

Note that I'm including portion sizes for the calories here. While in most restaurants the portion size is determined for you, you're on your own here, so I want you to get a good idea of how much you should dish out.

Top Picks

Salad dressings and croutons (for the make-your-own salad bar):

- Cucumber Dressing (80 calories/2 tablespoons)
- Fat Free Honey Mustard Dressing (45 calories/2 tablespoons)
- Fat Free Italian Dressing (20 calories/2 tablespoons)
- Garlic Parmesan Seasoned Croutons, low fat (40 calories/5 pieces)

TIP: If you're going to have croutons, consider them your starch and forgo the bread.

Signature Prepared Salads:

Many of these salads sound as though they'd be oily or mayonnaisey, but they're actually made with low-fat recipes.

- Aunt Doris' Red Pepper Slaw (70 calories/½ cup)
- Carrot Raisin Salad (90 calories/½ cup)
- German Potato Salad (120 calories/½ cup)
- Mandarin Noodles Salad with Broccoli (120 calories/½ cup)
- Marinated Summer Vegetables Salad (80 calories/½ cup)
- Morrocan Marinated Vegetables Salad (90 calories/½ cup)
- Oriental Ginger Slaw with Krab (70 calories/½ cup)
- Southern Dill Potato Salad (120 calories/½ cup)
- Summer Barley Salad with Black Beans (110 calories/½ cup)
- Tomato Cucumber Marinade Salad (80 calories/½ cup)

Fresh-Tossed Salads:
- Mediterranean Salad (150 calories/1 cup)
- Watercress and Orange Salad (90 calories/1 cup)
- Wonton Chicken Happiness (150 calories/1 cup)

Soups and Chili:
- Big Chunk Chicken Noodle (160 calories/1 cup)
- Butternut Squash Soup (140 calories/1 cup)
- Chicken Tortilla Soup with Jalapeño Chiles and Tomatoes (100 calories/1 cup)
- Deep Kettle House Chili, low fat (230 calories/1 cup)
- El Paso Lime and Chicken Soup (160 calories/1 cup)
- French Onion Soup (110 calories/1 cup)
- Garden Fresh Vegetable Soup (110 calories/1 cup)
- Hungarian Vegetable Soup (120 calories/1 cup)
- Living on the Veg Soup (90 calories/1 cup)
- Sweet Tomato Onion Soup (110 calories/1 cup)
- Three Bean Turkey Chili (140 calories/1 cup)
- Tomato Parmesan and Vegetable Soup (120 calories/1 cup)
- Vegetable Medley Soup (90 calories/1 cup)

Hot Tossed Pastas:
- Garden Vegetable with Meatballs (270 calories/ 1 cup)
- Italian Vegetable Beef (270 calories/1 cup)
- Lemon Cream and Asparagus (230 calories/1 cup)
- Oriental Green Bean and Noodles (240 calories/ 1 cup)
- Vegetable Ragu (250 calories/1 cup)
- Vegetarian Marinara with Basil (260 calories/1 cup)

Muffins and Breads:
- Apple Cinnamon Bran Muffin (80 calories)
- Buttermilk Cornbread (140 calories)
- Chile Corn Muffin (140 calories)
- Cranberry Orange Bran Muffin (80 calories)
- Garlic Parmesan Focaccia, low fat (100 calories)
- Indian Grain Bread (200 calories)

Not on the Program
Salad Dressings:
- Balsamic Vinaigrette (180 calories/2 tablespoons)
- Basil Vinaigrette (160 calories/2 tablespoons)
- Parmesan Pepper Cream Dressing (160 calories/ 2 tablespoons)

Signature Prepared Salads:
Calorie-wise, most of these don't seem too bad, but most of them have more than 11 grams of fat (some of it saturated), and when you consider that each serving is only ½ cup, that's too much.

- Cape Cod Spinach with Walnuts (170 calories/ ½ cup)
- Carrot Ginger Salad with Herb Vinaigrette (150 calories/ ½ cup)
- Dijon Potato Salad (150 calories/ ½ cup)
- Joan's Broccoli Madness Salad (180 calories/½ cup)
- Old-Fashioned Macaroni Salad with Ham (180 calories/ ½ cup)

- Shrimp and Seafood Shells (200 calories/ ½ cup)
- Tuna Tarragon Salad (240 calories/ ½ cup)
- Wild Rice and Chicken Salad (300 calories/ ½ cup)
- Zesty Chicken Salad (300 calories/ ½ cup)

Fresh Tossed Salads:
- Caesar Salad Asiago (190 calories/1 cup)
- Country French Salad with Bacon (210 calories/ 1 cup)
- Italian Sub Salad with Turkey and Salami (260 calories/1 cup)
- Pesto Orzo Salad with Pine Nuts (220 calories/ 1 cup)

Soups and Chilis:
- Baked Potato and Cheese with Bacon Soup (290 calories/1 cup)
- Black Bean Sausage Fling (350 calories/1 cup)
- Chicken Got Smoked (350 calories/1 cup)
- Cream of Mushroom Soup (290 calories/1 cup)
- Irish Potato Leek Soup (260 calories/1 cup)
- Make Room for Mushroom Soup (240 calories/ 1 cup)
- Not Skimpy on the Shrimpy (290 calories/1 cup)
- Shrimp Bisque (300 calories/1 cup)
- Toot Your Horn for Crab and Corn Soup (290 calories/1 cup)

Hot Tossed Pastas:
- Beef Stroganoff (340 calories/1 cup)
- Creamy Bruschetta (360 calories/1 cup)
- Fettuccine Alfredo (390 calories/1 cup)
- Nutty Mushroom (390 calories/1 cup)
- Smoked Salmon and Dill (360 calories/1 cup)
- Southwestern Alfredo Pasta (350 calories/1 cup)

Muffins and Breads:
- Big Blue Blueberry Muffin (310 calories)
- Black Forest Muffin (230 calories)
- French Quarter Praline Muffin (290 calories)

SPAGHETTI WAREHOUSE

www.meatballs.com

Traditional Italian-American dishes make up most of the menu here, which means there are lots of cream sauces, breaded and fried meats, and cheesy pastas. Stay away from anything with "Parmigiana" in the title, and stick with the very plain dishes.

Top Picks

- Tossed Salad
- Minestrone Soup
- Wedding Soup
- Spaghetti with Tomato Sauce, Tomato Sauce and Fresh Mushrooms, or Marinara Sauce—A feature on the Spaghetti Warehouse menu allows you to add grilled chicken and vegetables to your pasta, a nice idea.
- Chicken Alfredo Without the Alfredo—This would be a great dish if it wasn't accompanied by creamy pasta Alfredo. See if you can get them to substitute pasta with marinara sauce.

Not on the Program

- Calamari
- Lasagne and Chicken Parmigiana platter
- Turin Trio—Lasagne, Chicken Parmigiana, *and* Fettucine Alfredo, all on one plate.
- Baked Penne

STEAK 'N SHAKE

www.steaknshake.com

It might seem funny to go to Steak 'n Shake and have neither a steakburger (the item it's famous for) nor a shake. But if you can resist the restaurant's classics, there are a few other things on the menu that will be a lot better for you.

Top Picks

- Deluxe Garden Salad with Reduced Calorie

Ranch or Fat Free Golden Italian Dressing—Hold the cheese.
- Chicken Chef Salad—Ditto.
- Grilled Chicken Breast Sandwich
- Cottage cheese
- Soup—Provided it's not a creamy soup.

Breakfast
- Eggs and Toast—The eggs here always come with some kind of meat, but you can surely get them with nothing more than toast.
- Raisin Bran
- English Muffin

Not on the Program
- Triple Steakburger
- Any of the "melts"
- Chili 5 Way
- Fish Dinner—It's fried.

Breakfast
- Country Scrambler
- Strawberry French Toast

SUBWAY ★

www.subway.com

If you have seen any of Subway's television ads, you know that this chain prides itself on trying to help people lose weight. Its objective is to squash the notion that fast food is synonymous with "fat" food, and I think it's done a pretty good job of getting the message across. Sure, there are some things on the menu I'd advise you not to order, but there are a number of items in what Subway calls the "Under 6" category ("6" meaning 6 grams of fat). This category includes seven submarine sandwiches, which I think is particularly admirable since subs are typically some of the most fattening sandwiches going. Subway also has some healthful salads, adding to the nutritious selections. Some restaurants have so few healthy offerings that it's easy to get tired of going there, but you can eat at Subway often without having to order the same thing again and again.

Top Picks
Under 6 Sandwiches:
- 6" Ham (290 calories)
- 6" Roast Beef (290 calories)
- 6" Roasted Chicken Breast (320 calories)
- 6" Subway Club (320 calories)
- 6" Turkey Breast (280 calories)
- 6" Turkey Breast and Ham (290 calories)
- 6" Veggie Delite (230 calories)

Select Sandwiches:
- 6" Sweet Onion Chicken Teriyaki (380 calories)
- 6" Honey Mustard Ham (310 calories)
- 6" Red Wine Vinaigrette club (350 calories)

TIP: Opt for the honey oat bread, which has an extra gram of fiber.

Deli Sandwiches:
- Ham (210 calories)
- Roast Beef (220 calories)
- Turkey Breast (220 calories)

TIP: As Subway is happy to point out, if you prefer the Classic Sub you can order it without cheese and oil and it will be 72 calories and 7 grams of fat lighter.

Salads:
- Ham (110 calories)
- Roast Beef (120 calories)
- Subway Club (150 calories)
- Turkey Breast and Ham (120 calories)
- Veggie Delite (50 calories)

Soups:
- Roasted Chicken Noodle (90 calories)
- Vegetable Beef (90 calories)
- Minestrone (70 calories)
- Tomato Bisque (90 calories)

Not on the Program
Sandwiches:
- 6" Meatball (530 calories)
- 6" B.M.T. (480 calories)
- 6" Tuna (450 calories)
- 6" Dijon Horseradish Melt (470 calories)

Salads:
- Meatball Salad (320 calories)
- B.M.T. Salad (280 calories)

Soups:
- Cream of Potato with Bacon (210 calories)
- Cheese with Ham and Bacon (230 calories)
- Potato Cheese Chowder (210 calories)
- Brown and Wild Rice with Chicken (190 calories)
- Chili con Carne (310 calories)

TACO BELL

www.tacobell.com

As one of the first of its kind, Taco Bell set the stage for fast-food Mexican restaurants. To keep up with the times, it has changed its menu, though most of the newer items it's incorporated are not health-conscious. Still, it has a few offerings that aren't too bad, and I'm hoping that, like some other fast-food chains, it will add more nutritious offerings in the future.

Top Picks
- Soft Taco—Chicken (190 calories)
- Gordita Nacho Cheese—Chicken (270 calories)
- Bean Burrito (370 calories)

- Fiesta Burrito—Chicken (370 calories)
- Zesty Chicken Border Bowl without dressing (500 calories)—Use one of the many salsas Taco Bell offers.

Not on the Program
- Double Decker Taco Supreme (380 calories)
- Chalupas (350–430 calories)
- Grilled Stuft Burrito—Beef (730 calories)
- Zesty Chicken Border Bowl with dressing (730 calories)

TACO JOHN'S

www.tacojohns.com

There isn't a wealth of healthy dishes on Taco John's menu, but there certainly are enough good choices to satisfy your needs. One nice thing is that it offers tostadas that don't have a zillion calories, which they normally do. If you are smart about ordering, you can even extend the healthy offerings. For instance, the Chicken Festiva Salad with dressing is very high in fat and calories. But without the dressing, it's a reasonable choice and you can use salsa instead of vinaigrette to give it some added flavor. Look for these types of dietary loopholes and you'll do fine here.

Top Picks
- Chicken Softshell Taco (200 calories)
- Bean Burrito (380 calories)
- Bean Tostada (160 calories)
- Tostada (200 calories)
- Chicken Festiva Salad without dressing (390 calories)—See if you can also get them to leave off the cheese.
- Mexican Rice (250 calories)

Not on the Program
- Double Enchilada (750 calories)
- El Grande Burrito (730 calories)

- Sierra Taco—Beef (500 calories)
- Chicken Festiva Salad with Dressing (720 calories)
- Potato Olés (530 calories)

TACO TIME

www.tacotime.com

Here are three words to remember when you're eating at Taco Time: Hold the cheese. If you can get them to leave the cheese out of dishes like burritos and salads, your meal won't be half bad. The chain has a fairly limited menu, which means that the healthful offerings are limited too, but there are a couple of things that will work for you—even better if you can get them *sin queso.*

Top Picks
- Soft Bean Burrito (380 calories)
- Chicken and Black Bean Burrito (400 calories)
- Soft Taco (316 calories)
- Chicken Taco Salad (370 calories)
- Mexi-Rice (159 calories)

Not on the Program
- Big Juan Burrito—Beef (640 calories)
- Tostada Salad (628 calories)
- Taco Cheeseburger (633 calories)

TOGO'S

www.togos.com

When ordering here, keep in mind that the sandwiches come in two sizes. You should opt for the smaller one and, since the sandwiches are made to order, request that cheese and fatty sauces be left off your order. Although sandwiches are the specialty here, look beyond them, too—there are several good choices that don't come between bread.

Top Picks

- Black Bean Soup
- Chicken Noodle Soup
- Chili
- Turkey Sandwich—Hold the cheese and mayo, add vegetables.
- Avocado and Turkey Sandwich—It's not the lowest-calorie choice, but because avocado is a healthy fat, it's a nutritious sandwich.
- Roasted Chicken Sandwich
- Albacore Tuna Sandwich—They make it with light mayonnaise.
- Farmer's Market Salad—With the Low Fat Balsamic Vinaigrette.

Not on the Program

- Sicilian Chicken Sandwich—It comes with cream sauce and provolone.
- Avocado and Cheese Sandwich
- Meatballs in Zesty Tomato Sauce Sandwich

TONY ROMA'S ★

www.tonyromas.com

At first glance, you might not expect Tony Roma's to have many healthy choices. It is, after all, known for its barbecued ribs and deep-fried onion loaf. But fortunately for us, there are also plenty of grilled items and some simple vegetable side dishes on the menu. If you're looking for a place that will satisfy diners who are decidedly not on the program and those who are, this is a great choice.

Top Picks

- Marinated Chicken Grill
- BBQ Half Chicken—Request all white meat and remove the skin before eating.
- Grilled Shrimp Skewers—Have them leave off the lemon butter.

- Fish of the Day
- Grilled Chicken Salad
- Baked Potato
- Corn on the Cob

Not on the Program
- Potato Skins
- Potato Soup
- Chicken Tenderloin Platter
- Ribs
- Buffalo Chicken Sandwich

WENDY'S

www.wendys.com

With the introduction of its line of salads, Wendy's has contributed to making fast-food restaurants a safer place for those of us who want a nutritious meal. It's great to know that you don't have to be stuck with the same old limited choices of the past.

Top Picks
- Mandarin Chicken Salad (150 calories)—Add 130 calories if you mix in the roasted almonds, 60 calories for crispy noodles, and 250 calories for the sesame dressing.
- Spring Mix Salad (180 calories)—Add 130 calories for the honey roasted pecans, 190 calories for the house vinaigrette.
- Side Salad (35 calories)

TIP: Wendy's also has dressings that are lower in calories—fat-free French style (80 calories/packet), low-fat honey mustard (110 calories/packet), and reduced-fat creamy ranch (100 calories/packet).

- Grilled Chicken Sandwich (300 calories)
- Jr. Hamburger (270 calories)
- Baked Potato, plain (310 calories)
- Chili, small (200 calories)

Not on the Program
- Big Bacon Classic (570 calories)
- Chicken Club Sandwich (470 calories)
- Taco Supremo Salad with the works (670 calories)

WHATABURGER

www.whataburger.com

The motto of this burger spot is "Just like you like it." It says it's committed to customizing anything on the menu to suit its customers, so take advantage of the fact. Ask them to hold the cheese and fatty sauces. It's great to know that they'll oblige.

Top Picks
- Grilled Chicken Fajita Taco (363 calories)
- Grilled Chicken Sandwich, small bun, no oil on bun (334 calories)
- Whataburger Special Request, small bun, no oil on bun (427 calories)
- Garden Salad with Low Fat Ranch or Low Fat Vinaigrette (83–114 calories)

Not on the Program
- Triple Meat Whataburger (1,107 calories)
- Grilled Chicken Salad with Cheddar Cheese and Bacon (472 calories)
- Whatachick'n Sandwich (523 calories)

WHITE CASTLE

www.whitecastle.com

One of the oldest (if not *the* oldest) fast-food restaurants, White Castle claims to have made the hamburger an American icon. That's a dubious achievement, to be sure, but I'll give White Castle this: it's shown restraint in this age of the megahamburger by sticking to its 2.5-inch square patty. Of course, some people eat piles of the burgers, but the point is that if you want a reasonably sized burger (as those of us on the program do), you can get it here. At other places you may have to order the regular, cut it in two, then use extreme willpower not to eat the other half. But not here. Just order a regular Slyder, as White Castle calls them, and you needn't torture yourself.

Top Picks
- Hamburger (140 calories)
- Fish Sandwich (180 calories)
- Chicken Sandwich (190 calories)

TIP: If you find the White Castle burgers too small to eat just one, order a second and forgo the bun.

Not on the Program
- Bacon Cheeseburger (200 calories)
- Onion Chips (420 calories)
- Onion Rings (600 calories)

WIENERSCHNITZEL

www.wienerschnitzel.com

The menu at this hot dog chain is rather small, but Wienerschnitzel nonetheless has gone the extra mile and included a Healthy Choice Dog on the menu. That's a step in the right direction.

Top Picks
- Healthy Choice Mustard Dog—This has only 4 grams of fat, great for a hot dog.
- Healthy Choice Chili Dog—This one weighs in with 6 grams of fat.

Not on the Program
- Bacon Ranch Chicken Sandwich
- Corn Dog

YOSHINOYA ★

www.yoshinoyausa.com

Yoshinoya is a rarity: a chain that serves Japanese fast food. In doing so, it aims to make fast food a healthier proposition, and, for the most part, it succeeds. It is, for instance, one of the few places where you can get a big bowl of vegetables over rice for a quick lunch. Naturally, Yoshinoya offers a number of indulgent dishes as well, but if you stick to those that aren't fried, you'll do well here.

Top Picks

- Teriyaki Chicken Bowl—If you ask, they'll serve the chicken skinless.
- Vegetable Bowl
- Beef Bowl with Vegetables—According to the company literature, ounce for ounce, this dish has half the fat content of a typical fast-food burger.
- Chicken Salad
- Garden Salad

Not on the Program

- Breaded Shrimp Bowl
- Salmon Bowl—The fish is fried.
- Tempura Bowl
- Sesame Wings

Index

R

About the Author

Bob Greene is an exercise physiologist and certified personal trainer specializing in fitness, metabolism, and weight loss. He has been a guest on *The Oprah Winfrey Show*. He is also a contributing writer and editor for *O The Oprah Magazine,* and writes on health and fitness for Oprah.com. Greene is the best-selling author of *Make the Connection, Get With the Program!, The Get With the Program! Daily Journal,* and *The Get With the Program! Guide to Good Eating.*

You can visit Bob Greene at his website,
www.getwiththeprogram.org